OR
okas

Health and the Global Environment

Health and the Global Environment

Ross Hume Hall

Polity Press

Copyright © Ross Hume Hall 1990

First published 1990 by Polity Press in association with Basil Blackwell

Editorial Office:
Polity Press, 65 Bridge Street,
Cambridge CB2 1UR, UK

Marketing and Production:
Basil Blackwell Ltd
108 Cowley Road, Oxford OX4 1JF, UK

Essex County Library

ISBN 0 7456 0559 1

British Library Cataloguing in Publication Data
A CIP catalogue record for this book is available from the British Library.

Typeset in 10 on 12 pt Garamond by Photo-graphics Typesetters, Honiton, Devon
Printed in Great Britain by Billing & Sons Ltd, Worcester

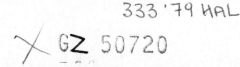

Contents

Acknowledgements

I could not have written the book without the help of others, and I owe my many colleagues in both the environmental and health sectors a debt of gratitude for the information and ideas they freely shared with me. It is impossible to mention all of them by name, but there is one person who deserves a special mention: my partner, Anne. We share a common interest in health and the environment. To her I owe the most.

R.H.H.

Introduction

This book is based on a straightforward premise: that our personal health depends on the natural environment. It is a premise we live with every breath, every sip of water, every bite of food. It is a premise that shows up in the unease over acid rain, global warming, ozone erosion, toxic dumps and contaminated water. It follows that we would wish to protect the quality of our environment – if for no other reason – to protect our health, our very lives. And in fact the driving force behind moves to correct environmental ills is the perceived threat to human health. Indeed, this force not only drives, but also shapes the way in which environmental policy is developed and the way in which particular environmental actions are taken.

This book argues that if we are going to deal effectively with global ills we must realize that the priority given to human health shapes environmental action to a considerable extent, and not necessarily positively. The reason for this lies in how threats to health are perceived. Whose perception of the threat determines how an environmental action, if any, will be launched? The answer – and this is part of the book's premise – is that perception of threats to health from the environment is filtered through the political and bureaucratic processes of our environmental and health institutions.

The environmental actions that emerge are slow, lacking in sufficient momentum to match the ever faster-moving global problems that threaten to overrun us. It is like a race in which our competitor runs on pavement and we run in mud.

The book explores why the drive for environmental protection and its promise of health is so blunted. And herein lies a paradox. The public is willing to support measures in pursuit of personal health, but although the environment–health connection is generally recognized, the health budget of nations is invested in a vast health-care system – in the United States the cost of the system is fast approaching 15 per cent of the Gross National Product. In contrast, only minuscule sums are invested in environmental protection. And this allocation of resources is not confined to money: the intelligence and zeal with which we pursue health through hospitals, doctors and medical research is overwhelmingly superior to anything mounted in the environmental sector.

It is a paradox that I saw in my teaching experience. The most articulate, the brightest of undergraduate students headed straight into medical school or medical research. Of the hundreds of students who passed through my hands, the fingers of one hand tally those who have made a career of trying to improve the environment. There is nothing intrinsically wrong with improving medical care, but my students missed the point that an improved environment would prevent many of the ills the health-care system has to try to cure.

The paradox in the environment–health connection became even more conspicuous in my environmental work. Although my main job was doing medical research and teaching biochemistry to students in medicine, nursing and the sciences, I was drawn into the environmental movement, both in citizen groups and as a scientific adviser to Canada's Minister of Environment.

I entered the movement as a scientist with a research background in cancer and toxic chemicals, but I soon found myself not so much serving as an expert in these subjects, as dealing with the grittiness of environmental policy-making. It was then I realized that almost every environmental decision was driven in some way by a concern for human health. Politicians may express concern over wildlife or preserving natural beauty, but wildlife and the environment seldom provoke decisions for their own sake.

What particularly struck me about the governmental bureaucracy of the environment was that nowhere was an expert on human health to be found. The bureaucrats had no expertise in these matters, although decisions – often non-decisions – affecting human health were made daily. The Canadian government does indeed have expertise in human health – a gargantuan health bureaucracy and a budget some forty times larger than the environmental budget. But this health bureaucracy has little time for, or interest in, the environment.

Yet I found that government health bureaucrats and the health-care systems at large – and this is part of the paradox – had a decisive role in how decisions in the environmental sector were made. The principle on which that influence operates can be summed up in one word: cure. The health-care system operates on a basis of waiting until a patient walks through the door with a complaint and then dealing with the problem. This is what hospitals and doctors are set up to do. And it is through the cure approach and all its ramifications that the health-care system exerts its strongest leverage over the environmental sector.

My purpose in writing the book, however, was to go beyond an exploration of the leverage of the health-care system. You will find running through the chapters a case for dropping the cure approach to environmental ills and taking a hairpin turn to prevention. The idea of a preventive approach, of course, has been urged by many, including the World Commission on Environment and Development. Gro Harlem Brundtland, Prime Minister of Norway and the Commission's chairperson, and her commissioners underscored the need for a change in approach: 'We are unanimous in our conviction that the security, well being and very survival of the planet depend on such changes, now.'

But how does society translate the phrase 'preventive approach' into action? A case for prevention in the chapters that follow is built on the premise that concern for human health drives environmental action and that a healthy environment is a desirable framework for protecting the public's health. The book uses that premise as a springboard towards resolution of the contradictions in the environment–health connection that block a move towards prevention and a healthier environment.

But in making a case for prevention, I have had to face the fact that environmental and health institutions operate in two different worlds. For this reason the book is divided into two parts: the first five chapters centre on the health-care institutions from an environmental perspective: the remaining chapters expand into environmental issues from the global public health perspective.

My main sources of information are conversations with a large number of people working in the health and environmental fields, the technical literature in both fields and constant observation of how health and environmental issues unfold. The book is intended for a general audience concerned with environmental and health issues and with the long-term betterment – as Lester Brown of the Worldwatch Institute puts it – of the human prospect.

Part I

Health Care and Attitudes Towards the Environment

1

Prevention: A Case for Dropping the One-cause/One-effect Model

The idea of a relation between health and the environment is far from new. The ancient Greeks entrusted their health to a beautiful goddess, Hygeia, who promoted good health through a sound personal environment. Our word, hygiene, comes from this lady. But Hygeia demanded a certain commitment from the individual in order to achieve good health, a commitment that many Greeks found hard to make. So they turned to other gods who promised health through medicine and hospitals. Human nature has not changed and in modern times people continue to neglect or abuse their bodies believing that even if this leads to illness, the doctor will heal them. René Dubos commented on this facet of human nature in his book, *Mirage of Health*: 'Men as a rule find it easier to depend on healers than to attempt the more difficult task of living wisely.'[1]

Some thirty years after Dubos wrote those words, Brundtland picked up his theme of living wisely. She remarked on the folly of human societies conducting their affairs without heeding the way their actions lead to environmental degradation – as if humans themselves had no connection with the environment. She and her Commission found that, although attempts are made to clean up and protect the environment, these attempts can be characterized at best as feeble. She cited a general backing off of government from coming to grips with the complexities of environmental problems and she was particularly harsh on the institutions that have been been created to deal with environmental problems: 'Scientists bring to our attention urgent but complex problems bearing on our very survival. We respond by demanding more details, and by assigning the problems to institutions ill equipped to cope with them.'[2]

Clearly, in Brundtland's view, governments have failed to organize an appropriate response to environmental threats; they have failed to set up the appropriate institutions for social planning, research and action. Governments may be making an effort to deal with environmental problems, but the effort, in the Commission's view, is too meagre to prevent a downward slide in the state of the environment. But, although the World Commission outlines environmental woes in naked detail, it does not offer detailed solutions. What it does is to throw out a challenge to world societies to design new courses of action that will halt and reverse the slide.

In accepting the challenge, one could say: 'We need to continue what we are doing now but to do it harder.' Or one could say: 'Scrap the present approach and apply a different one.' Our present approach is akin to that of Dubos's sufferers – we wait until the environmental problems roll over us, then we take action. It is cure-after-the-fact. The issue can be illustrated with an anecdote.

Imagine visiting a river and hearing a drowning person shouting for help. You, a strong swimmer, leap in, but you no sooner pull this person on to the shore when another struggling victim floats into view. You rescue this second person only to be confronted with a shout from yet another drowning person. You decide this situation makes no sense, so you rush upstream to find a bully throwing people into the water.

When you rescue people from the water you make use of your superior swimming skills: that is what curative medicine does. You could teach the drowning people how to swim – if they will listen: that is what health promotion does. Or you could deal with the bully and prevent people from being thrown in the water. Prevention requires going to the source of the problem and fixing it.

So that brings us to the crux of the challenge: how do you switch the course of action from cure-after-the-fact to prevention? It is not a case of playing the game harder: we have to change the playing field. The biggest barrier to making the switch to prevention lies in the health-care systems of the industrialized nations. These official systems – the hospitals, the medical societies, the government health bureaucracies, the drug companies with their vested interest in cure – have a profound influence on how an environmental problem is defined and whether or not any priority should be given to tackling the problem.

I should hasten to add that this is not a malevolent influence, deliberately aimed to thwart solutions of environmental problems; rather, the influence is a fallout as these health bodies go about their business of curing the ill. The net effect of the influence on environmental action, however, is analogous to that of a dragging anchor on a ship trying to sail. Moreover, the influence is difficult to recognize, still more to confront. Because the influence is indirect, you can not very well go to a medical meeting and complain to surgeons and drug manufacturers that they are a drag on environmental policy.

One of the tasks of this book is to bring out ways in which the health-care system directs environmental decision-making. For the moment, I concentrate on one of the principal ways: motivation. The health-care system influences environmental policy both in the intensity of motivation and in its direction. Motivation is critical; there has to be a driving force, an upsurge of public indignation and support for any corrective programme. If you ask people why they support a particular environmental programme, most will answer that they are concerned for their health and that of their children. It is this concern for human health that drives environmental policy and decision-making, and it is through this very human desire to be fit and healthy that the impact of the health-care system is felt most.

I will go on to elaborate on this thesis, but before I do, it is important that we distinguish between curative and preventive approaches to environmental problem-solving. The distinction is critical in understanding why Brundtland, her commissioners and many environmentalists believe the switch to prevention is overdue.

Smog: Add-on Cure or Prevention?

What does environmental prevention mean? You might respond that there are lots of anti-pollution programmes under way; if they are not working so well, why not apply more diligence? In any event, anti-pollution programmes seem to be a form of prevention, so how does a preventive approach differ from what is already being done?

Consider a well-defined environmental issue: city smog. Although most cities of the world share the smog problem, Los Angeles has become the most publicized example of a city doomed to life in a permanent caustic cloud. Los Angeles also attracts publicity because it became one of the first cities in the world to try to fix its smog. Twenty years ago the state and city instituted a number of measure to ease the smoggy burden, and in fact, clean air laws since enacted at the federal level in the United States and in other countries had their trials in Los Angeles.

Los Angeles diagnosed its main problem as automobile emissions. The internal combustion engines of cars and trucks emit unburned hydrocarbons (gasoline) and nitrogen oxides. These two substances in the presence of sunlight react to form a mixture of over 100 different irritating, caustic chemicals that hang in the streets. Clean-up policy concentrated on forcing car manufacturers to install catalytic converters that transform the exhaust gases into less polluting gases. In addition, hydrocarbon evaporation from fuel spills was closely regulated.

Progress was dramatic and the smog level in Los Angeles and in other cities dropped; but now, two decades later, the smog in Los Angeles is worse than it was before the clean-air laws were introduced. Air quality in the city on half the days of 1988 fell below the acceptable standard set by the Clean Air Act. What does this mean for the health of the city's residents?

Doctors for years thought that air pollution was a problem only for individuals with asthma or emphysema. But now, according to Thomas Godar, president of the American Lung Association, healthy adults and children who exercise moderately when the air quality falls below government standard can suffer impaired lung function and other respiratory problems.[3] This health problem is not peculiar to Los Angeles. Many major cities in both North America and Europe have many days a year when air quality is as bad as it is in Los Angeles.

So, after twenty years of clean-air laws and anti-pollution measures, why is air quality worse than it was in the 1960s? Part of the answer is that the air envelope of Los Angeles now has to absorb the exhaust gases of more cars and trucks, driving more miles than ever. Although each vehicle emits less pollution than formerly, the total exhaust injected into the envelope is greater. Automotive engineers, encouraged by politicians, are searching diligently for a solution by designing even more efficient and less polluting engines. But reduction of exhaust pollution can only go so far if the object is still an engine that runs. In any event, critics say, the search for more efficient design only staves off the inevitable eventual bumping up against the finite air envelope as more people drive more cars. Los Angeles is enacting other measures, such as banning all aerosol spray cans, but against the principal cause of the smog – cars and trucks – anti-pollution measures are what can be defined as add-on or end-of-tail-pipe measures, trying to cope with exhaust gases *after they are produced.*

A long-term, preventive solution takes a more radical view: eliminate the internal combustion engine. It is the only way to go, according to William Chameides, a geophysicist at the Georgia Institute of Technology, who studies smog formation: 'In the long run I believe we must

get away from all forms of combustion and perhaps go to electric
vehicles. Every other approach is just a stopgap remedy.'⁴

It is one thing to install a catalytic converter in your automobile. It
is quite another to give up the gas-burning vehicle altogether and go for
an electric one. Can you imagine the social and political problems that
would be created if the internal combustion engine was phased out? Oil
companies would go the way manufacturers of steam locomotives went
in the 1950s. Car manufacturers would have to give up their investment
in gasoline and diesel engines. Jobs would be lost. Where would the
electricity come from? Merely contemplating the social upheaval is
enough to discourage a politician from even considering such a course.
It is the kind of environmental solution that Senator Albert Gore Jr of
the US Congress, an advocate for a co-operative global agenda on
environmental issues, calls 'almost unimaginably difficult.'⁵

We have to realize that when we talk of prevention, we are talking of
major changes in use of the underlying technology in society – in this
case transportation technology. The change does not have to mean a
lowering of living standards: just a different way of doing things with a
whole new set of opportunities. It is the transition, however, that makes
politicians blanch. It is like contemplating having a tooth drilled without
anaesthetic. Is the repaired and useful tooth going to be worth the pain?
On the other hand, a little novocaine eases the transition from decayed
tooth to mended tooth. Politicians and business leaders fear the preventive approach because we have never bothered to create the institutions
or government policies – the novocaine – to ease society's transition.

Maurice Strong, a member of the Brundtland Commission, speaking
of the dependence of the economy on a healthy environment, said: 'If
we want industry to operate in a way that is sustainable for society as
a whole we need a system of incentives and penalties that make it
profitable for them to do that.'⁶

It is the absence of such transition policies and institutions that Brundtland identified when she talked of institutions 'ill equipped' to solve
environmental problems. Thus we have environmental agencies that try
to enforce clean-air laws and automotive engineers who design and build
better internal combustion engines, but these agencies and these engineers
are ill equipped to solve the problem of city smog.

The issue of air pollution and the internal combustion engine is just
one of a large catalogue of environmental issues. But it illustrates the
difference between trying to fix a problem by adding on – in this case
by tail-pipe controls – and going to the root of the issue and adopting
a preventive strategy. The add-on approach is a technical solution. It
requires no social engineering apart from persuading people to drive

smaller cars and pay for catalytic converters. In the politicians' view, however, the add-on, technical approach avoids the political pain of asking businesses and people to adopt a new style of life.

Human Health Concerns Motivate Environmental Clean-up

What stops us from adopting a preventive approach to solving environmental issues? Gutless politicians? It is handy to blame the politicians, but the answer lies far deeper, in the attitudes that society as a whole has towards the environment. We have to ask ourselves: What is the motivation for making any attempt at all to control pollution? Los Angeles is a vibrant, economically sound community. Most residents go about their lives seemingly unaffected by the pollution. The citizens may feel they have already undertaken extensive anti-pollution measures; what would their motivation be for undertaking more?

Motivation is critical to finding solutions to environmental degradation, and we might judge from the growing list of environmental problems reported in the media that our collective motivation is stunted. We then have to ask what has been the main motivating force for the steps taken so far to clean up pollution? Has it been a love of wildlife, a love of natural beauty, a feeling that we humans are the stewards of the environment? Each of these feelings plays a role – but a minor one. The major motivating force is concern for human health.

Self-interest obviously underlies this motivation, but nevertheless, it is what drives policy-makers to action. People have a strong sense of self and are more likely to demand action when their own health and well-being are threatened. It is easier to drive public policy with human health than with environmental protection. Position papers of organizations, such as the World Health Organization (WHO), that document the human health effects of a polluted environment, have far more clout with scientists and policy-makers than those of environmental agencies that merely outline environmental degradation.

In other words, if a health body gets behind a recommendation for environmental action something is more likely to happen than if a purely environmental organization urges action. This is not to say that just having the support of health bodies automatically launches environmental action; it is that such action is more likely to take place if that support exists.

Environmental legislation – clean air laws, water quality laws, waste dump laws – are all defined and administered with human health as the end-point. The criteria for the success of these laws are measured in terms of the removal or minimization of threats to human health. Rarely does one find environmental legislation or regulation based on the health and well-being of other species. It is fair to say that the body of environmental law is designed to protect human health; the environment is protected in as much as there is some perceived benefit to humans. There is no law that covers the sanctity of the environment in its own right.

This narrow view of what constitutes harm to the environment angers many environmentalists. It means that they frequently are unable to interest governments in correcting gross environmental abuse because they are unable to convince officials of a link between the abuse and a threat to humans. As it is, governments seldom act unless the threat is well defined and a reasonably simple remedy can be applied. You see the operation of such practical politics in governments' response to compelling evidence of climate instability. Two threats to climate stability have recently emerged: the erosion of the ozone shield and an excess of carbon dioxide in the atmosphere. In one case you have decisive action; in the other, waffling.

A layer of ozone in the stratosphere prevents the sun's ultraviolet radiation from reaching the earth's surface. Man-made chemicals, the chlorofluorocarbons (CFCs), a million metric tons a year of them, are reaching the stratosphere and destroying the ozone, allowing more ultraviolet radiation to penetrate. Threats to health are clear: increased incidence of cataracts, a lowering of immune defences and, above all, an increase in skin cancer. The US National Academy of Sciences estimates that a drop in ozone levels of only 1 per cent could cause 10,000 more cases of cancer in the United States alone. Reaction to the health threat has been swift: already an international agreement to phase out CFCs has been ratified by thirty-nine nations, including members of the EEC, the United States and Canada.

Carbon dioxide is another story. It is produced by combustion of oil and coal and by the burning of forests. It is the chief gas that atmospheric scientists say is going to raise global temperature by 1–5°C by the year 2050 (the process known as the greenhouse effect). Although much is written and leading politicians are saying something should be done about global warming, no consensus on action has emerged. One reason is the absence of a clearly defined threat to human health. There are, of course, indirect threats – heat stroke or lack of food due to drought, but these are vague and debatable. The whole problem, in fact, seems too vague to politicians, the threats too speculative; moreover, further research may show there isn't a problem after all. Senator Gore sums up this attitude, prevalent among his congressional colleagues: 'Well maybe we won't really have to face up to it.'[7]

This leisurely attitude contrasts with the view of many atmospheric scientists who believe that global warming is not just imminent; it has started. The greenhouse effect is only one of the global stresses that endanger the viability of the planet, all demanding decisive action at the political level. 'Time is not on our side,' said Lester Brown. 'We have years, not decades to turn the situation around, and even then there is no guarantee that we will be able to reverse the trends that are undermining the human prospect.'[8]

And Edward Goldsmith, editor of the *Ecologist*, spells out why the world environmental situation has suddenly become so critical: 'more destruction has been wrought to the fragile fabric of the biosphere during the last 40 years, since global development has really got underway, than during the preceding two or three million years of the human experience on this planet.'[9]

Environmentalists like Brown and Goldsmith conjure up a vision of world ecodisaster in terms of expanding deserts, deforestation, soil erosion and extinguished wildlife. That vision, however, is not translated into a threat to human health in a way that puts fire in the bellies of political leaders. Governments, and the way they act, express a different vision of the state of the world from Brown. The government vision is straightforward: politicians and officials have to see a direct and clear impact of the environmental degradation on the health of people. If this threat is not clearly defined, they feel they can declare in good conscience: 'no problem'. This narrow vision, like a pencil-thin flashlight, enables political leaders to see a threat to health in the erosion of the ozone layer, but is incapable of floodlighting the threat of increased atmospheric carbon dioxide. So why is the vision so narrowly focused? Let us turn to the advisers who define human health threats from the environment.

A Medical Vision of Environmental Threats

Designers of environmental programmes – the politicians and public officials – are not experts in human health, so they turn to medical experts for advice on whether or not there is a health threat, and if there is, how serious it is. Medical experts, in turn, advise only in the terms they know how to use, in the terms of their own medical experience and training: paradoxically, an experience and a training that pays scant heed to environmental causes of human illness. Medical education teaches doctors what to do when a patient walks or is carried through the clinic door. Doctors are taught to diagnose the problem and then proceed with a treatment. There is little or nothing in this training to provoke an interest in the reasons for the illness. Doctors are trained as healers.

This medical disinterest in causes of illness pervades the whole health-care system. This is not to say there are no public health officials or individual doctors interested in causes of illness, but the weight of medical practice and money spent is directed at cure. Although much of human disease is incurable, money is spent either trying to cure it or searching for the cure. It is an anomaly that prompted Lewis Thomas, a physician and chairman of the Memorial Hospital, New York, to write: 'The trouble with medicine today is that we simply do not know enough; we are still a largely ignorant profession, faced by an array of illnesses that we do not really understand, unable to do much beyond trying to make the right diagnosis.'[10]

In spite of the ignorance that Thomas talks of, there is no concerted effort among the medical community to find ways to avoid disease. Their research resources – which are formidable – are applied to inventing new drugs, developing the technology of organ transplant, searching for a cure for cancer. Very little of that research effort is earmarked for developing the means to prevent disease. I will be expanding on this thought in some detail in later chapters. At the moment I simply wish to make the point that, although some research into environmental causes of human illness is done, the sophistication of this research is the equivalent of a grass skirt compared to the *haute couture* of cure-directed medical research.

The net result is that the idea of what constitutes an environmental threat to health has advanced very little since the middle of the nineteenth century. In fact, the medical thinking you find in environmental medicine is rooted in the public health successes of that period. For an example, we can go back in time to John Snow, a London physician, who in 1854 was faced with a cholera epidemic. Snow felt intuitively there was some connection between the disease and the city water the citizens got from a pump on Broad Street. This was about the time bacteria were disco-vered and the idea of providing clean drinking water was just emerging. A decisive man, Snow removed the handle from the pump and was gratified to find, shortly thereafter, that the epidemic subsided.

The nineteenth-century discovery of the link between bacteria and disease established a medical mindset of a cause – a germ – and the disease it caused, that is, one cause, one disease. This style of thinking continues today and is the style that medical advisers use to define environmental threats to human health. You can see the one-cause/one-effect thinking at work in a ruckus over an apple spray.

Apples: Hazardous to Your Health?

The ruckus illustrates how the health-care system defines the human health end-point for a specific environmental situation. The chemical, Alar,[11] is sprayed by apple-growers on their trees to strengthen stems, preventing apples from falling before they ripen. Growers using it find they get more uniform ripening and less bruising and can pick the whole crop at one time. But the chemical persists in the apples, penetrating about a centimetre into the flesh where it cannot be removed by washing or peeling. The chemical has government approval even though some ten years ago Alar was shown to cause cancer in laboratory animals.

US government spokesmen said that the residues in apples, apple juice and apple sauce were too low to affect humans. But apple juice and sauce are popular foods with youngsters. The Natural Resources Defense Council, a group based in Washington DC, did some calculations showing that, because children drink a lot more juice than adults and because of their small body size, they received, in effect, large enough doses of Alar to push their cancer risk to a much higher level – 250 times that of an adult.[12] The initial reaction of government health agencies was to repeat public statements that Alar poses no threat to children, and that, in any event, the cancer threat is offset by the nutritional value of the juice and sauce. 'There is no scientific data presently available that convinces us that there should be any restriction of use for at least Alar,' Bonnie Fox-McIntyre, an official of Health and Welfare Canada was quoted as saying.[13]

But Fox-McIntyre ignored the larger point made by the Natural Resources Defense Council: that growers chose from over 100 different chemical sprays and that a grower, on average, used between six and twenty different pesticides on a crop. The Council's concern was not only the Alar, but residues of all the other chemicals in apple juice and sauce. But government officials, unwilling to think in terms of more than one chemical at a time, restricted their response to Alar, and having judged the cancer risk from this one chemical as acceptable, they declared the apples safe for children. When Fox-McIntyre says she has no data she is right: the government never tests mixtures of chemical residues for their potential to harm. Yet it is the mixtures which enter the human consumer.

You see the ghost of the nineteenth century in the response of the health officials to this situation – the one-cause/one-effect definition of what constitutes an environmental problem. This perception of an environmental issue brings out two features that deserve emphasizing.

First, the health threat: officials assessed one chemical residue in the apples and one effect – the potential to cause one disease, cancer. They made their judgement as if no other chemical residues existed, as if no other harm to health was possible. Second, the environment: the apple orchards were just a backdrop, a source of a chemical contaminant. The health officials ignored the fact that during the spraying only a small fraction of the chemicals actually landed on the apples, the rest wafting away into the environment. The potential for harm extends beyond humans. There is no sense of the continuity and totality of the environment.

The Natural Resources Defense Council estimated that 6,200 children of the current pre-school population of the United States will get cancer at some point in their lives because of having consumed apple juice and sauce contaminated with Alar. The health-care system is well suited to caring for the cancer cases when they arise, but it is not well suited to preventing the cases from arising. Hospitals and all the other institutions of the health-care system see themselves far removed from apple orchards and the growing practices of farmers. One would not expect doctors and hospital administrators to worry about growing apples.

Yet, paradoxically, because of their way of thinking about environmental threats to health and because human health is the end-point of environmental action, the professionals of the health-care system have a powerful influence on the way farmers are licensed to spray toxic chemicals and the fruit is allowed to convey the residues to consumers. The whole issue of environmental protection is carried out in a way that fits the perceptions of these health professionals. They are interested only in the effects of environmental contamination, in this case residues of a chemical spray; they are not interested in the causes of the contamination. The health-care system has no mechanism for asking: Do farmers have to use chemical sprays to obtain crops?

One has to ask if this is the best institutional arrangement for integrating two interests that seem to be in competition: growing fruit profitably and eating fruit without being poisoned. It is an end-of-tail-pipe approach similar to that used to deal with automobile exhausts. The present arrangement allows the health-care system to detach the health issue from the growing of apples and to determine the safety of what is on and in the apples. It is another example of the cure-after-the-fact approach. A preventive approach would integrate the method of growing apples into the whole issue of environment and human health; but there are no institutional mechanisms for working out such an integration.

A Case for Dropping the One-cause/One-effect Model

Rearranging institutional mechanisms by themselves, however, would be insufficient; there has to be conceptual change in the approach to environmental issues, a dropping of the one-cause/one-effect model and its replacement with integrative thinking. The case of the Alar-contaminated apples may seem quite simple, but it illustrates how we isolate an environmental issue from the broader horizon of the integration of trees and humans into the scheme of the world ecosystem.

James Lovelock, author of the book *Gaia: A New Look at Life on Earth*,[14] is one individual who sees the larger horizon. He studies the broad interactions of living organisms with the geological and atmospheric forces of earth and describes the human place on the planet in these terms: 'I see the world as a living organism of which we are part: not the owner, not the tenant, not even a passenger on that obsolete metaphor "Spaceship Earth".'[15]

If one thinks in Lovelock's terms – that our lives are an integral part of the life of the planet – then to maintain health, we must avoid interfering with the broad interactions of this earthly oganism. Think of the world as a house. All the hospitals and high medical technology will not save our health and well-being if the environmental walls and roof crumble.

Lovelock's global perspective seems far removed from apples and the threat of cancer, but if our institutional arrangements for growing fruit and for assessing safety took into account the broad global horizon then issues such as toxic chemical residues on fruit would not arise. The political reality, of course, is that our institutions do not work that way. The reality is that the health-care system dominates the institutions we set up to protect the environment. The end-point for that protection is human health and the interpretation of a threat to health is filtered through the one-cause/one-effect model.

The defining of most environmental problems in one-cause/one-effect terms is one of the gravest weaknesses of this medical model. How do you grapple with the issue of global warming in such terms? The answer, of course, is that you cannot, and what happens is that, if the problem cannot be defined in one-on-one terms, officially it does not exist. Thus we have many government officials downplaying the threat of global warming because they see no direct connection with a health issue, or downplaying the health threat from drinking Alar-contaminated apple juice at age five because this isolated risk in their view is trivial.[16]

I give these examples to illustrate the power of medical thinking in defining environmental issues and courses of action (although the course of action quite often is to do nothing). More fundamentally, what this power does is to lock environmental policy and action into trying to cure problems after they arise. It is this after-the-fact approach, as mentioned earlier, that the Brundtland Commission found unworkable. It is an approach outmatched by the problems that face human society. 'The rate of change is outstripping the ability of scientific disciplines and our current capabilities to assess and advise,' said the Commission.[17]

Brown, Brundtland, Gore, Lovelock and many others describe these environmental problems in terms of cathedral-like complexity: all we see at the moment is a blurred rectangular shape. We know the cathedral is there and that it has an intricate structure, but we are unable to make out the details. The challenge is to deal with these complex, blurred problems using the preventive approach. To start, we have to learn how to define the problems and solutions in a preventive way. Brundtland and her commissioners call for a switch to prevention by going to the source of environmental problems: 'The time has come to break out of past patterns. Attempts to maintain social and ecological stability through old approaches to development and environmental protection will increase instability. Security must be sought through change.'[18]

The remaining chapters of this book are designed to make a case for breaking out of the pattern of defining environmental threats to human health in terms of the one-cause/one-effect model and to demonstrate how the problem can be redefined from a preventive point of view. This first part probes from an environmental perspective the attitudes of health professionals and the commercial and political forces that shape the operation of the health-care system; and, by extension, how these attitudes shape environmental policy. Any plea for a comprehensive, preventive approach to environmental protection has to acknowledge this almost overpowering influence. The second part examines how this influence with its one-cause/one-effect model limits the effectiveness of environmental action.

2

A Biomedical Model of Health

The question of why environmental policy is so locked into its one-cause/one-effect model may seem remote from a London ambulance driver. But if we are to trace the origins of the model and address the question of its grip first on the health-care system and second on how that system applies the model to environmental issues, the ambulance driver is a good place to start. This driver had considerable insight into the health consequences of a health-care system centred on cure. One of the medical team working with patients brought in by the driver was Susan Rosenthal, a recently graduated medical doctor. She told me of the driver's comments about a bronchitic patient he had just delivered to the hospital. The driver described the home environment of the patient: the mouldy wallpaper, inadequate heat and poorly prepared, unfinished meal. He remarked that the state provides the means to treat this man's repeated bouts of bronchitis, but is incapable of organizing the means to deal with the man's home environment. 'You see,' she said, 'the ambulance driver was powerless to influence health policy in an illness-centred, health-care system.'[1]

Indeed, the response to an increasing number of patients with chronic breathing problems is the demand for more hospitals, the training of more staff, the manufacturing of more drugs and machines. Bronchitic patients can be brought to the hospital, have their pained breathing relieved and then be sent home until the next attack. The medical staff are specialists in treating bronchitis, not in dealing with mouldy wallpaper. And would one expect them to be? Rosenthal's point was that, because the health-care system is so illness-centred, governments funnel public funds and resources almost exclusively into the treatment of illness.

As the ambulance driver noted, resources that could help prevent bronchitis are not forthcoming; the system, in effect, waits until the illness strikes, then attempts a cure. What are the origins of this bias? If you thought of the entire health-care system as an organism, you would identify the medical profession with the brain. It is how doctors think about the human body in sickness and health and how they see the body in relation to its environment that determine the attitudes of the system as a whole. How doctors think is critical to an understanding of how the health-care system operates, why it funnels resources into treatment and cure and how this policy affects environmental policy negatively.

From the point of view of the sick patient it is hard to think of faults in the health-care system. The availability of doctors and medical care is a blessing. But for the sake of the argument in this book we stand away from the system and look at the total perspective, and what we see is a paradox. Although the resources of the health-care system are focused on illness and its cure, restoration of health is not always achieved, particularly for serious and chronic illness. Much serious illness, in fact, is incurable, according to Trevor Hancock, a public health physician with the Toronto Board of Health and a critic of the cure bias of the health-care system. Hancock cites several studies conducted by the Canadian and United States governments that conclude 'that the health-care system plays a minor role in determining our state of health.'[2]

The implication behind Hancock's remark is that since a lot of serious disease is incurable, a better approach is to prevent it. It is a paradox that our health-care system delivers cure and not prevention when, in fact, so much illness is incurable. Is it fair, however, to put the blame for this one-sided approach on the shoulders of doctors? They may be the brain of the health-care system, but they are the product of a tradition that itself is shaped by many social and commercial forces. It is worth examining this tradition to see how indelible it is and how slowly it changes. A broader social issue then emerges: whether we should expect doctors to include prevention in their thinking or whether an additional class of health professional is needed, one able to put humans into their broad social and environmental context and to understand the role of those contextual factors in prevention of human affliction.

Social Transformation of Medicine from
Prevention to Cure

The word prevention, in its broadest health sense, is what today we would call environmental protection. And if you go back 100 years, that was what preventive health meant. The greatest proportion of public money in the field of health care in the nineteenth century was actually earmarked for prevention of disease. The engineering of sanitary sewers and public water mains was a major factor in wiping out tuberculosis, cholera and typhoid, major causes of death during the nineteenth century. These infectious diseases have given way to cancer and heart disease as this century's symbols of human frailty and susceptibility to disease. But can we really extend nineteenth-century emphasis on prevention to such complex ills as cancer and heart disease? After all, the nineteenth-century engineers had only to eliminate the disease-causing microbes from the public environment. It is easy to say that now, but consider the problem of maintaining health from the perspective of a nineteenth-century health official. Cholera and typhoid were as mysterious and profound to them as cancer and heart disease are to us. The big difference is that they sought solutions to their health problems through prevention; we seek solutions through cure.

The transformation of public policy from a health-care system centred on prevention to one centred on doctors and their curative powers coincided with the rise of scientific medicine and the development of medical technology. The diagnosis of diseases using complex and expensive machines and the transplantation of organs through complex surgery are skills that only doctors possess. It gives them a mystique and a power in the health-care hierarchy denied everyone else.

The cure bias of doctors also removes any interest the health-care system might have in environmental issues. Such issues, for the most part, are deemed irrelevant to the public's health, a dismissal that has a profound effect on environmental policy. This is a subject I will take up later.

The Biomedical Model and the Mechanical
Image of Life

Do doctors really have that much influence on the health-care system? They make up only a small fraction of what we loosely define as that system: for every doctor there are some twenty other workers, from ambulance drivers, nurses and computer clerks to drug researchers, pharmacy clerks and government bureaucrats. The health-care system includes a vast array of activities having to do with human health, from home care to hospitals. There is no activity, however, that is not directed in some way by doctors: their decisions generate 95 per cent of all health expenditures. The whole system revolves around how doctors think and practise their medicine. All these workers, in fact, share a common image of human health. But the doctors, because of their authority and visibility, shape and project an image of how the human body works, how it falls into disease and how it should be cured.

In other words, doctors have a conceptual framework within which they define health and sickness, a framework which defines how they will go about maintaining the health of the population. This conceptual framework is called by some the *biomedical model* and that is the term that I use.

The biomedical model obviously promotes cure but the conceptual image it promotes is more fundamental. It projects the idea of the human body as a machine. Perhaps the rawest expression of this image was given by the French geneticist, Jacques Monod. Winner of the 1965 Nobel Prize for physiology and medicine, Monod wrote: 'anything can be reduced to simple, obvious mechanical interactions. The cell is a machine; the animal is a machine; man is a machine.'[3]

Monod believed that, although we do not yet know all the parts or all the interactions of the human body, we will some day; and that we will be able to catalogue the human body as we now catalogue the parts of a motor car. The image of the machine does indeed conjure up an assembly of parts, all meshing with each other, each essential to the performance of the machine. Break or displace a part and, depending on how critical the part is, performance falters. To maintain performance, therefore, one need only identify the malfunctioning part and do something about it.

A machine image of the human body invites a curative approach. You are given a body at birth; it has to last a lifetime. Suppose you were given a motor car at birth, and the car had to last a lifetime. You would depend on the skill of the mechanics to diagnose and repair the inevitable failure of parts and systems. The analogy is not at all far-fetched; doctors see themselves as experts at diagnosing malfunctioning parts of the human body and making the necessary repairs or cure. The mechanical image encourages extreme specialization.

A colleague who once complained of an intestinal problem found himself examined by one doctor who examined only his upper intestinal tract. Then a second doctor examined his lower tract, and finally a third doctor did his middle. Three separate visits and examinations, three separate bills.

There is an alternative image to the mechanical one and its associated specialization: an image that portrays the human body as a complex whole in which every part of the body is touched by any one illness. It is an image that portrays the body, not in mechanical isolation, but in close relationship with its social and natural environment. Although some doctors and health workers champion this image, the critical question is: What drives the health-care system? The answer is: the mechanical image of the biomedical model, and moreover, this image is so strongly held that it allows no room for an alternative, more holistic view of human health.

You see the mechanical view of the individual expressed in many ways. Thomas Preston, a cardiologist at the University of Washington, Seattle, tells how this view can distort the patient–doctor relationship.[4] He admitted to the hospital a 60-year-old woman with an erratic heart-beat. It was not an emergency, but Preston wanted to try a new drug and keep her under observation. The lady arrived at 3.00 p.m., the drug was administered and she was resting comfortably. She took a sleeping pill and at midnight fell into a deep sleep. As is usual in large teaching hospitals, the head doctor admits and is responsible for the patient, but medical care is delivered by house doctors, residents and interns. At 2.30 a.m. the resident and intern on the ward entered the patient's room, woke her up, took a personal history and did a complete physical exam. She was not amused.

Preston found out about the incident next morning and asked the two young doctors, 'What if she hadn't been in hospital? Would you have gone to her home and wakened her at 2.30 am?'

They replied that it was not proper to leave her 'not worked up' and that they had only done what they were supposed to do. Preston commented that what the two doctors had actually done was to pay heed to their professional standards rather than to the comfort of the patient. He went on to say that a few years back when these same two doctors began their medical studies, 'they would have been appalled at an act so discourteous and unhelpful from the patient's perspective.' But as the two advanced through the medical subculture they shifted their loyalty from patient to doctor. In other words, they were learning to do the right thing by the biomedical model, or as Preston called it, by *professional standards*. It is this fixation, he adds, that sets the tone for a physician's behaviour throughout his or her career.

A Reductionist View of the Human Body

From what we know about the interactive relations of living organisms in the world ecosystem, the mechanical image of the human body seems out of joint. Such an image leaves scant room for human feelings, the rhythms of life and especially the ecological linkages of each of us to all other living species, from apples to lake trout to tropical forests. Our present interest in this matter lies in how the mechanical image affects the practice of medicine and how it carries over into public attitudes towards the living world. The reason for the interest is that public support for environmental protection depends a great deal on the dominant image the public has of environmental processes. A mechanical image of the environment invites the add-on or cure approach to environmental problems. The contrasting, ecological view of the world environment invites the preventive approach.

Is the dominant image of the world ecosystem the mechanical image doctors have of the living body? It is worth exploring this question in more detail. First, a little history, because the biomedical model has its origin in seventeenth-century science. A predecessor of Jacques Monod, the French philosopher and mathematician René Descartes (1596–1650), tried to establish a general theory to explain the universe, based on physics and mechanics. He included all living organisms in his theory, believing that they were all merely machines. Even the human body was a machine, powered by the beat of the heart, fed by the food carried in the blood. Descartes believed that to understand the whole machine one must identify and understand all the parts. This philosophical legacy flourishes in scientific thinking over 300 years later – expressed in Monod's words quoted above – and in the practice of today's scientific medicine.

You often see Descartes' legacy expressed in the term *scientific reductionism*. By this view, the system under study is too large and complex to understand so it is reduced to ever smaller units, the implication being that understanding of the whole through observing its parts is thus possible. For instance, the amount of cholesterol in one's blood – a part of the human body – is used in scientific medicine as an indicator of degenerative disease of the heart.

Reductionism fosters analysis and much of today's medical science is, in fact, analysis – of blood cholesterol levels, X-rays and the amount of dioxin in drinking water. Diagnosis of an illness is analysis, the ability to analyse a sick body, to arrive at a conclusion. The opposite of analysis is synthesis. Doctors certainly perform a synthesis in the diagnosis when they put together a pattern of analytical findings, but in a broader sense synthetic skills are surpisingly weak. Although we have sophisticated laboratory procedures for analysing cholesterol in blood and dioxin in drinking water, for example, our understanding of heart degeneration is sketchy and interpretation of the health effects of dioxin remains a guess. Synthesis implies reaching for a broad interpretation of findings and that is where the weakness lies. Synthesis, in effect, is the opposite of reductionism; it implies wholeness.

Let us take the point about synthesis further. When we talk of a whole we need to define it. If we start with the human body, cholesterol is one of its parts. On the other hand, if we start with world ecology a human being is one of its parts. Thus, if we are interested in human health, we need to work in both directions. It is essential to know something of the body parts, including cholesterol, and how they work (reductionism); and it is essential to know how humans connect to their environment (synthesis).

But reductionism fosters observation and thinking in only one direction, towards smaller units. Human health is observed and treated in isolation from its environment. You see this in one of the more popular images of scientific medicine, a group of doctors standing around a horizontal body, dead or alive, and carrying out some form of analysis or diagnosis. It is the classic picture of the human body isolated.

The belief that human illness can be understood by studying the human body all by itself makes it difficult for medical doctors to think about the relation of human beings to their environment. For the most part, they do not feel that such relationships are important. Such an attitude finds expression in the 2.30 a.m. awakening of a 60-year-old lady for a physical exam. Science, although embracing reductionism, also has room for synthesis, an outlook at the broad connections. But some branches of science, physics for instance, are better than others at balancing reductionism and synthesis; others remain strongly biased towards analysis or reductionism. Medical practice (and its biomedical model) is one of those.

The Rise of the Biomedical Model

I do not wish to leave the impression that scientific reductionism is a negative force. It is a powerful scientific approach that gives us a lot of insight into how the human body works. And its successes, in effect, give a stamp of authority to the biomedical model. To gain some insight into why the model has retained such a tenacious hold we should consider the early rise of modern medical science. It is a big success story for Descartes' reductionism.

The one scientific event that set modern medicine in motion was the development of the compound microscope. The microscope had been invented by Anton van Leeuwenhoek about the time Descartes was active, but it was not strong enough to show the cells of animal tissues. The compound version, invented in Germany in the early nineteenth century, greatly increased resolving power, enabling details of the cells that make up animal tissues to be seen. Until that time, what doctors knew about the human body were the organs and bones they saw with their naked eyes. The compound microscope gave them the ability to reduce the size of what they saw. Where hitherto they saw a liver, they now saw details of the trillion or so cells that make up a human liver. The workings of the liver were revealed in a way hitherto impossible.

There is more to science than having a tool, and it was the brilliance and forcefulness of one individual, Rudolph Virchow (1821–1902), that took the microscope and transformed the practice of medicine. Virchow, a German medical doctor, looked at the tissues of sick people and noticed changes in the structure of the cells. The changes in different people with the same ailment were the same and Virchow realized that he had discovered a reliable method for classifying disease. Before Virchow, doctors classified their patients as having a fever or a stomach ache: what we now call symptoms. There are many causes of a fever but the early doctors could only deal with the fever. Virchow was able to see under those symptoms and discern that many different illnesses give rise to the same symptoms. He had a much better understanding of why the patient was sick.

Virchow's scientific research had enormous impact on how doctors were trained in medical school and how they thought about sick people. Doctors no longer talked about ill patients; they talked about patients with typhoid, or tuberculosis, or liver cancer. Virchow's science also had a less visible, but nevertheless just as profound effect on the medical thinking of the nineteenth century. It confirmed the power of Descartes' scientific reductionism: total understanding of the human body and its illnesses could be rationally based on measurable scientific and clinical data.

But whereas scientists and doctors fervently believe in the objectivity of measurements, they tend to forget that the measurements are limited by the tools available. Virchow's science of diagnosis was developed on the basis of an ability to reduce the human body into small units, the cells, and measure their state. Modern science, of course, reduces the human body to parts much smaller than the cells, to the genes and the molecules that make up cells. But although modern medical science has made enormous advances, its underlying philosophy is still that of Descartes. It is analogous to a train starting on a journey. Virchow started the train on its way, since when it has indeed gone far; but it is still on the same track, and the train's direction is limited to that of the track.

Virchow was one of many gifted nineteenth-century medical scientists. His contemporary in France, Louis Pasteur (1822–95), also applied the compound microscope to the study of how microbes cause disease. Pasteur's view of microscopic organisms fitted with the mechanistic view of the human body. The microbes turned a switch that threw the body into a disease state. Get rid of the microbes and the body is switched back to good health, none the worse for the experience (providing, of course, one survived the infection).

Pasteur and Virchow thought in both scientific directions, analysis and synthesis. Yet while they are well remembered for their mechanistic science, they are less well remembered for their sensitivity to the broader issues of public health. Microbes, in Pasteur's view, should be considered only one of many causes of disease: how the microbes are carried and how a person becomes infected were just as important. Virchow spent much of his time in politics. Elected a member of the Berlin City Council in 1851, he campaigned successfully for safe drinking water and ample sewer lines. Virchow claimed that political and socio-economic factors were significant causes of disease and that, therefore, disease was amenable to elimination through social change.

This macro view of humans and their environment contrasted with the micro view of human tissue seen through the compound microscope, but Pasteur and Virchow were able to think about and integrate both views into a total picture of environment, human health and disease. The macro view withered away, however, as our industrial societies moved into the twentieth century. Twentieth-century scientific medicine embraced only the micro, or body-as-machine, view of how the human body works and fails.

It is this view that underpins the biomedical model, framing the way doctors think and act. It is a view that stresses finding out what is wrong with a human body and fixing the problem. Thus we come back to a London ambulance driver lamenting the British health-care system's inability to prevent disease.

Educating a Doctor

So just how does the biomedical model affect the way a doctor thinks and acts? The most direct way of answering that question is to trace how the model conditions medical students. Medical schools are society's prime instrument for shaping the biomedical model and defending it against heresies, such as chiropractic, homoeopathy and herbal medicine. You will not find a course labelled 'Biomedical Model 101' in any medical school. The model is not taught as such, but it is meticulously instilled into students through the teaching environment. Here is how one student, albeit an unusual student, described his experience.

Melvin Konner was a PhD anthropologist with field experience among the !Kung San bushmen of the Kalahari desert when he entered Harvard Medical School at the age of thirty-five. He went through the four-year medical programme, a member of the tribe of medical novitiates, yet distant from them. He carefully kept notes of what happened along the way and how he reacted to what happened, and, on graduation, he wrote a book about his anthropological field trip: *Becoming a Doctor: A Journey of Initiation in Medical School.*[5]

Konner's book describes one year of his experience, the third of the programme. This is the year when embryonic doctors meet their first living patients. The first and second years at Harvard, as at most US medical schools, are devoted to mastering the basics of medical science, biochemistry, physiology, anatomy and cellular pathology. The students spend all their time in classrooms and laboratories, never coming into contact with the world of doctoring.

But in his third year, Konner was expected to start applying his basic science to the sick. The first place a novice doctor meets sick people is in a hospital. Konner found himself thrust into the bewildering world of hospital medicine, a world peopled with very sick people – many of them dying – none of whom he ever saw wearing street clothes. Where he expected compassion, he found detachment and ribald humour. Where he expected time to spend with patients, he found visits with each fleeting. Where he expected to lay hands on people he found himself laying hands on machines. He saw his patients through CT scans, MRI images[6] and computer printouts of blood analyses. His hospital world was populated by hordes of technicians, aides, nurses. The population, much to Konner's surprise, did not include senior staff. Rarely did the world-renowned medical professors of Harvard appear in his life. His teachers were interns and residents, students with a year or two more experience than himself. But it was a strong learning experience and through it all, he describes with satisfaction the bursts of clinical insight when his book theory and practice came together.

The insights that Konner described, howere, were insights into what was wrong with his patients: the ability to diagnose. The four-year medical programme is designed to teach students how to diagnose, that is, how to classify the set of symptoms the patient presents into a recognized disease. This approach lies at the heart of the biomedical model. Medical wisdom holds that you can not treat a problem unless you know what the problem is. It is necessary to determine what part or parts of the body are not working properly and then afterwards do something about these defective parts.

Very little of the medical students' time is spent learning treatments, because once a diagnosis is made; a specified treatment is automatic. Moreover, much of the treatment is administered by nurses, therapists and technicians – or by the patients themselves (e.g. taking a pill). Diagnosis is the pre-eminent skill in the medical world, and only doctors are legally empowered to practise it.

Konner went through his third year at Harvard Medical School in 1983/4. If he had waited a couple of years he could have been part of Harvard's New Pathways programme, which started in 1985. This programme takes about one fifth of each medical class and immerses the students in the traditional sciences and clinical art mixed with a patient-centred humanism. It is an attempt to foster the notion in budding doctors that their patients are not just bodies but individuals with worries and families, people who wear clothes and live and work somewhere.

The key to the Harvard programme is integration and an awareness that bodies are also people. The closest that most schools come to teaching this awareness is in medical ethics. Of the 126 medical schools in the United States, 112 offer a course in ethics, humanities or doctor–patient relationships; but these courses are wedged in between the students' science and clinical courses. Many students feel the courses have little to do with real medicine and tend to ignore them. The big difference with Harvard's New Pathways programme is that such courses are not separate; rather, the human side of medicine is built into the students' technical learning.

Students start working with patients at the outset. Much of their learning is self-directed and done in tutorial groups of five or six as opposed to sitting passively in large lecture theatres. The students are given more opportunity to challenge basic assumptions of medical care, and – the designers of the programme hope – will carry the challenging attitude with them throughout their professional life. The programme puts greater emphasis on the patient, not just in terms of high-technology treatments, but in forming an integrated picture of the behavioural, social, nutritional aspects of the medical problem. The goal of the programme is that the student sees the medical problem as a human being located in a network of family, work and environment.

The New Pathways programme has met mostly indifference or outright hostility in the medical world. Scientific medicine is so complex and bursting with new knowledge, critics feel, that any activity other than the teaching of science wastes student time. But to critics who say there is not enough time in the four-year curriculum for both science and humanism, Daniel Tosteson, Dean of Harvard Medical School, replies: 'To say that the New Pathways programme is developing more humane physicians at the expense of science-rooted competence would be wrong. We are after a better balance between the natural scientific, the social scientific and the humanities aspect of medicine.'[7]

The critics were not convinced. 'Science is the fundamental basis of medicine and there is no way we can diminish it,' said Richard Ross, Dean of Johns Hopkins Medical School.[8] Ross did not believe there was time to fit humanities courses into a medical curriculum of some 4,000 hours of lectures, laboratories and demonstrations. Henry Seidel, another Johns Hopkins medical official, added that society plays a larger role in shaping physicians' attitudes. 'Physicians should always be caring – I don't think that is an issue. But are we a caring society? All these programmes won't really matter unless society changes.'[9]

Tosteson defends the New Pathways programme as a response to a rapidly changing world. The public's sense of values is changing. There is a realization that much of the disease that afflicts modern populations is incurable and can only be managed. And then there is a technological explosion of knowledge related to human biology and health that we do not know how to handle. Medical professors admit that the standard medical curriculum with its limited time is like requiring the students to drink from a fire hose. Tosteson sees the New Pathways programme as an answer to the deluge, a way for the students to sort through new knowledge and develop the scholarly skills for keeping up with developments as they go through their careers.[10]

The debate within medical circles over medical education is obviously lively. Although it tends to focus on secondary issues of whether or not medical education is humane – a doctor can still adhere to the tenets of the biomedical model and not wake his patients up in the middle of the night – nevertheless, the debate shows a willingness on the part of many doctors to draw away from strict adherence to the biomedical model and to recognize that the human body does not function in isolation.

The directors of the Association of American Medical Colleges have been particularly vocal about the need for change. They believe that a changing society requires a different type of medical professional, and they backed up their beliefs with a report, entitled 'Physicians for the Twenty-First Century', which strongly recommends a switch to the Harvard-type programme.[11] Tosteson, though, is realistic about what will continue to happen in most medical schools because of the entrenched views of the medical education establishment (as expressed, for example, by the Johns Hopkins dean) and he does not expect any major shift. Nevertheless, there are medical schools that follow this integrated, self-directed learning format. McMaster University, Hamilton, Ontario, pioneered this type of programme starting in 1969. Rush, Southern Illinois and New Mexico medical schools in the United States have all adopted parts of this approach as have Maastricht (Holland), Ben Gurion (Israel) and Newcastle (Australia).

Life after Medical School

The New Pathways programme at Harvard and similar programmes in other universities, although shifting away from the exclusive science-based, traditional programmes, still stress cure, that is, diagnosing and solving the problems of sick people. Moreover, graduates of these programmes still have to function in a medical world set within the biomedical model. They must pass licensing exams that test their mechanistic knowledge of the human body. They come under the powerful influence of the established practice of medicine: hospitals, drug companies, medical societies. All these influences in the end may be more powerful than any changes in the curriculum.

There is another compelling factor that makes it difficult to put a more human face on the practice of medicine: specialization. Scientific medicine generates an enormous amount of factual knowledge. The human mind is limited by its nature in the amount of detail it can grasp, and as medical science generates ever more details, doctors keep splintering into ever narrower areas of speciality. Medical education, especially in the United States, turns out doctors who, after their initial undergraduate medical programme, go on to specialize and sub-specialize. Some eight-five per cent of doctors in the United States are trained in a medical speciality. There is, in the view of some, a glut of specialists: too many, chasing too little disease. 'There are few echocardiograms in search of a cardiologist to read them, there is only a rare belch wanting a gastroenterologist, and there is not a single even slightly plugged coronary that does not have three specialists waiting in the wings.'[12] The words of a stand-up comic? No; those of Robert Petersdorf, president of the Association of American Medical Colleges. Petersdorf took over the presidency in 1986 following a twenty-year period of rapid growth in the physical plant of medical education in the United States. Existing medical colleges expanded and forty new ones opened. Petersdorf feels that all these colleges are turning out far more doctors than the country is able to digest, or at least the wrong types of doctors. He is particularly critical of the over-emphasis on high-tech medicine and the excessive specialization that goes with it. He wants to reduce speciality training. It is easy for young doctors to specialize, he says, because the government pays for their speciality education, for as long as five years. Petersdorf would make less government money available, hoping to discourage young doctors from seeking the narrow training.

If, as Petersdorf suggests, there are more specialists than disorders to be treated, will that not encourage specialists to move into a more general practice? Events would suggest not.

Mather Menken and Cecil Sheps, neurologists at Rutgers Medical School, New Jersey, tell of how a glut of neurologists earns a livelihood. The number of patients with neurological diseases is fixed. Neurologists tend to spend more time, therefore, with each patient – good, you might say, time for a better doctor–patient relationship. But that time is spent subjecting the patient to a broader range of procedures and examinations – at greater cost to the patient – and to what end, say Menken and Sheps? 'It is not at all clear that this increased intensity in the use of procedures makes a crucial difference in outcome for all patients.'[13] Moreover, in their desire to maintain their patient load and income, neurologists start treating patients with lesser problems, patients who would be better treated by a general practitioner, rather than being subjected to a lucrative (to the neurologist) electromyogram for low back pain.

Dean Tosteson has a point: there is much entrenched in the education of doctors and in the practice of medicine that militates against an open view of human beings and their society. Thre is no incentive for young doctors not to specialize, and although there are medical spokespersons (invariably specialists themselves) who would like to see a shift in balance between high-tech, specialized doctors and those able to relate to patients and their environment, the shift is barely perceptible.

From the point of view of medical policy, it is the specialists who make the policy. The United States may have a higher proportion of medical specialists than other countries, but in all countries it is the specialists who occupy positions of prestige in medical societies and medical faculties and who dominate policy-making bodies. In spite of the talk of more humane teaching and practising, it is the specialists and their interpretation of the biomedical model that are likely to persist. It is an interpretation that attaches little importance to investigating and understanding the human–environment connection.

Cure versus Prevention: Asclepius versus Hygeia

George Washington was a robust 66-year-old when he went horseback riding one morning in the snow. On his return, he complained of a fever and a sore throat, went to bed and called his doctors. They wrapped a poultice around his neck, gave him a honey and vinegar gargle and over the next two days drained him of two and a half quarts of blood. His last words to his doctors before he died were, 'Pray take no trouble about me. Let me go quietly.'

Washington lived in the eighteenth century, an era when doctors felt compelled to do something. They believed, and their patients believed, that without some form of ministering they (the patients) would die. The range of treatments was not large: opium, strong purges for the bowels, cupping poultices and copious bleeding. It was a no-lose situation for doctors and their medicine. If the patient survived, the value of the treatment was proven. If the patient died, the illness was beyond the reach of medicine.

But early in the nineteenth century, these treatments were being challenged, and Pierre Louis, a French physician, in 1836 conducted what must have been one of the earliest attempts to prove whether or not a medical treatment really worked. He divided several patients with pneumonia into two groups; the patients in one were drained and cupped while the other group was left alone. Louis concluded: 'We infer that bloodletting has had very little influence on the progress of pneumonia.'[14] The studies of Louis and others showed that the medical heroics of the eighteenth century were of little value. The medical profession was devastated. The experiments, however, instilled a new belief among doctors: 'If you don't know what to do, don't do anything.' This radical switch in attitude occurred while Virchow, Pasteur and other scientists were laying the basis for scientific medicine. But while these researchers did a great deal to explain illness, they offered no new treatment. Physicians of the nineteenth century were astute enough to realize that if left alone, patients recovered from most illnesses.

Society's attitude towards the environment in the eighteenth and nineteenth centuries paralleled the physicians' attitudes towards the human body – in reverse. While eighteenth-century physicians believed their purges, bleedings and cuppings kept the population healthy, their cities rotted in the filth of garbage, sewage and unclean water. And while nineteenth-century physicians backed off intervening in people's biology, cities made great strides in providing clean water and dealing with sewage and garbage.

The situation is like a coin. When we turn the heads side up, the tails side is hidden, and when we turn the tails up, heads disappears. We see only one side at a time, either environment or medical intervention. The twentieth-century turn of the coin has put medical intervention and cure back in vogue.

Like eighteenth-century doctors, modern doctors find it difficult not to do anything. Melvin Konner discovered this fact on his initiation into hospital medicine: there are so many drugs, solutions and machines to apply to people. And in truth, many patients and their families will sue for malpractice if the doctor fails to inject or prescribe or connect a machine. Yet much modern doctoring is applied to incurable situations. Lewis Thomas notes simply: 'A great deal of the time and energy expended in a modern hospital is taken up by efforts to put off the endgame.'[15] According to Roger Evans, a health economist at the University of Washington, 30 per cent of expenditure on health care in the United States is spent on individuals who die within a year of initiation of their treatment.[16] Prevention, of course, cannot stave off human mortality, but the concept of prevention allows the rhythms of life to take their natural and dignified course.

This oscillation between seeking health through medical intervention and a less intrusive approach has been going on since the time of Hygeia and the ancient Greeks. Hygeia, the patroness of health through prudent living, ruled the lives of this ancient culture until the fifth century BC when a new God, Asclepius, displaced her. Asclepius, a handsome young man according to Greek legend, advocated the surgical use of the knife and the curative power of drugs. Belief in the powers of Asclepius led to the rise of a professional class of doctors. Not all Greeks were convinced of the wisdom of following Asclepius. Plato wrote in his *New Republic* that the need for many doctors and hospitals is the mark of a bad city. The alternation between Asclepius and Hygeia has continued throughout the centuries; we are currently under the power of Asclepius. Curiously, there is a rigidity to the Hygeia–Asclepius coin; we seem to be able to see only one face at a time. But you find that many critics of medical over-specialization and advocates of a more humane medicine are really advocating a balance between the two gods. If you are injured in a fire, it is nice to have a burn specialist available, and it is also nice to have a doctor who can help you prevent illness. Robert Spasoff, professor of preventive medicine at the University of Ottawa, however, sums up the view most doctors have of prevention: 'It's unexciting, it's not glamorous, it doesn't use fancy equipment or produce dramatic

3

Reinforcing the Image of the Human Body as a Machine

What kind of image does a magazine advertisement for the throat gargle Chloraseptic convey? The drug, manufactured by Eaton Laboratories, Norwich, NY, according to the advertisement, blocks the ninth cranial nerve, the nerve that telegraphs the brain that the throat is sore. The copy reads: 'You need it (the nerve) to tell you something's wrong. Once. But you don't need a constant reminder – Chloraseptic acts as an anesthetic so it actually helps block the pain impulses.'

The advertisement does not claim to cure the sore throat, but it does claim to cure you of the sore feeling. The mechanical image promoted here is that there is a single message route to the brain and that a drug – Chloraseptic – magically blasts this message route. There are many reasons why the throat may be sore – inflammation, infection, etc. – and the soreness is a symptom of a more fundamental problem not addressed in the advertisement. By promoting the cause-and-effect image of a sore throat and simple relief, the complex nature of sore throats is passed over.

This chapter is about the image that people have of their personal biology in health and sickness. The image can be summed up in the expression 'machine-like'. You can see that mechanical image coming through in the promotion of a seemingly innocuous sore throat remedy. It is not likely that many of us articulate such an image in so many words, but it shows up in the way we treat our bodies, or allow others to treat us with a drug. The act of taking a drug expresses the image of our body working like a machine, the sore throat or headache switched off by the chemical. In a broader sense, it is an expression of the cure-over-prevention biomedical model under which doctors are trained to operate and within which, in fact, the whole health-care system operates.

In the previous chapter I focused on the training of doctors as a way of identifying the mechanical images embedded in the delivery of health care. In this chapter the focus is on the proposition that most people, as consumers of health care, willingly subscribe to the machine-like image of their bodies. So what if they do? One could say that holding such an image is strictly a matter for the providers and consumers of health care, but my proposition is part of a broader thesis that the mechanical view of human biology extends to the world about. And as we shall see later, this view casts an obstructive shadow over environmental policy and actions.

But for now let us explore the proposition that the way doctors think is the way their patients think, or in other words, that the doctor's biomedical model has been adopted by the general public. In particular, let us explore it through the most common of all health-care actions – the taking of a drug.

Drugs as Magic Bullets

It is hard to come away from a visit to the doctor without a prescription for a drug. Doctors on average write one and a half prescriptions for every patient visit. The prescription symbolizes the doctor's power to diagnose the cause of the problem and to cure the problem with the drug. The drug may or may not affect the outcome of the problem – most minor illnesses, which account for the majority of visits to doctors, are self-correcting – but the individual feels that medical intervention has been necessary and successful, that the drug has switched him or her back to health.

It would seem that modern society is unable to survive without drugs. The average family in the USA collects fifty prescriptions a year. Every day, according to one survey, 65 per cent of the adult population of Britain take a doctor-prescribed drug.[1] These figures do not include the large number of remedies purchased without a prescription or over the counter (OTC). The ready swallowing of drugs – which are chemicals foreign to the body – is a continuing reaffirmation of faith in medical intervention and medical technology.

The image behind drug technology is one of drugs as magic bullets targeting the one cause of an illness. The idea behind the magic bullet is that it passes magically through the healthy parts of the body without causing damage, striking only that part of the body that is causing the health problem. It is an image of drugs that has been around since the end of the nineteenth century, an image that persists among doctors and the public today in spite of much evidence that drugs are not so magical, that a shotgun blast would be a more appropriate image. Drugs, in fact, are powerful interveners in one's biology and, like real bullets, are capable of doing great damage to healthy body systems.

The universal home remedy, aspirin (acetylsalicylic acid or ASA), on the market since 1899, has a range of actions, going beyond its relief of aches and fever. In many people, it can cause intestinal bleeding, impaired blood clotting, accelerated or depressed breathing and a general malaise. The heavy promotion of aspirin to the public does not indicate that any of these side-effects may occur. The advertising copy, in effect, perpetuates the image of aspirin as a magic bullet for aches and pains.

The idea of drugs as magic bullets, in view of our modern ecological understanding of how biological processes interact with each other, does seem simplistic. So it is worth our while spending some time examining why this image persists. There is an implication in this exploration: that there are alternative ways of viewing human biology and of dealing with human affliction. But these alternatives tend to get lost under the weight of what John Kenneth Galbraith called in economics the 'conventional wisdom of the system'. In our case conventional wisdom favours the machine-like view of the human body. Consider how conventional wisdom deals with a health problem common among middle-aged people – high blood pressure or, in the medical term, hypertension.

Hypertension: Drugs versus Environmental Factors

High blood pressure is an example of how belief in the magic bullet isolates thinking about a health problem. The magic bullet image encourages both doctor and patient to believe that this human ill can be treated in isolation from the social, economic and natural environment of the individual. The drug treatment, in effect, is carried out as if the individual were unconnected to these environments. Yet by paying some attention to these connections the need for drugs can vanish. Still, in spite of the alternative and in spite of the danger taking the drugs may pose, physicians favour the drug treatment.

Just what is hypertension, and why is it amenable to non-drug treatment? Mild to severe hypertension, which afflicts some 60 million Americans, is a symptom rather than a disease; it signifies some deep-seated disarrangement of one's biology. The exact nature and cause of the disarrangement are unknown, although there is a fair amount of information about the immediate reasons for the hypertension. One, for example, is hardening of the arteries: the arteries become less resilient, making it harder for the heart to pump blood. We know that this happens, but how does it start and why does it occur in some people and not in others? There is a lot of uncertainty.

Even mild hypertension increases the risk of a heart attack or stroke, so it is beneficial to the individual to bring blood pressure down. Treatment centres on the immediate causes, and a variety of drugs have been invented that minimize the effect of one or more factors; but none addresses the underlying body deterioration. A physician presented with an individual with hypertension will usually start by prescribing a diuretic. Diuretics cause frequent urination, eliminating sodium and excess body fluid. This eases the strain on the heart. But there is a problem; potassium is lost together with the sodium. Potassium is essential for nerve transmission and muscle contraction; excessive potassium loss can be fatal, causing the heart to stop beating. So doctors may prescribe a potassium supplement.

If the diuretic fails to work, the doctor can give a drug, called a beta-blocker, which interferes with nerve impulses to the heart and arteries. The net effect is that the heart beats less strongly and the arteries relax, reducing resistance to blood flow. If the beta-blockers fail to work, the patient can try a drug that interferes with calcium flow. Calcium is required for nerve stimulation of the muscles that surround arteries. The net effect again is to relax the arteries, decreasing the resistance to blood flow.

There are still more drugs in the physicians' armoury, such as alpha-agonists, which interfere with normal release of the hormone noradrenaline by the brain. Such interference also causes the heart to slow down. With so many drugs available, there are cases of patients (presumably with enthusiastic doctors) taking five different drugs, each several times a day. An aptitude for mathematics is almost a basic requirement to keep the pills and their times straight.

Do the pills work? An antihypertensive drug or some combination of such drugs can indeed lower blood pressure, but in spite of this, patients with hypertension have a higher incidence of heart disease than the general population. One study, by Michael H. Alderman of the Albert Einstein College of Medicine, New York, found that for many patients with mild hypertension drug therapy actually increased the risk of stroke or heart attack.[2] One reason for this apparent contradiction is that hypertension is only a symptom of deep-seated changes occurring in the patient's heart and arterial system, and the drugs do not really address these changes.

The drugs certainly do not cure hypertension and so an individual is going to have to take the drug or drugs for the rest of his or her life. Most of these drugs are new and the side-effects of decades of use are completely unknown. It was this fact that prompted Rose Stamler of the Department of Community Health and Preventive Medicine at Northwestern University Medical School, Chicago, to look for an alternative to the drugs.

Stamler and her colleagues made a study of patients with severe hypertension who had been taking drugs for five years previously.[3] The patients stopped taking the drugs and instead received counselling on a prudent diet. About a third of the patients lost an average of 4.5 kg in weight, and the group as a whole reduced their salt and alcohol intake. The study continued for four years, during which 40 per cent of the patients were able to maintain normal blood pressure without taking any drugs. Others in the group managed by taking lower doses of antihypertensive drugs than they had taken before entering the programme.

Stamler noted that the programme benefited the patients in two ways: their blood pressure was lower and they avoided unwanted side-effects of the drugs. The main point of the Stamler study is that an alternative to drug treatment works when you put the patient into the context of his environment, including his nutritional environment.

However, altering one's dietary habits requires commitment and willpower. Drugs, in contrast, have a psychological advantage for many people, because they require the patient to exercise no responsibility for the treatment; it is entirely in the hands of physicians and drug companies. The patients act like passive bodies, accepting whatever is done to them. Drug companies are banking on the lack of willpower and the strength of the magic bullet image among the 60 million Americans with high blood pressure. Although some doctors will advise their patients of the Stamler alternative, the drug companies obviously feel that the majority will not; the companies predict a doubling in prescriptions of antihypertensive drugs over the five-year period 1987–92, with an increase in sales value from $4.3 to $8.5 billion.[4]

The fact that antihypertensive drugs take preference over non-drug alternatives brings out another aspect of people's image of their bodies in health and illness. Individuals with hypertension are, in fact, fitting their personal biology to the style of drug therapy whereas the alternative fits the therapy to the realities of human biology.

One casualty in the ready acceptance of antihypertensives and indeed all drugs as magic bullets is loss of the sense that health is attainable by paying close attention to one's social and natural environments.

Educating Doctors about Drugs

The preferred treatment of high blood pressure with drugs brings out a facet of health-care that deserves spotlighting. Drugs are products of the chemical industry and the financial welfare of the industry lies in selling drugs. There is no money for drug companies in advising people on good eating habits. The commercial promotion of drugs is a powerful force in determining how the health-care system operates, and the industry has a strong financial stake in the image of drugs as magic bullets. It is that image that sells.

As mentioned above, there are two categories of commercial drugs: over-the-counter (OTC), available without prescription, and prescription drugs. Both categories are heavily promoted. You see the promotion of OTC drugs on TV and in journals. But you do not see the equally heavy promotion of prescription drugs to doctors through their professional journals and through direct calls at their offices. This promotion is more intense and more important to the drug industry than that for OTC drugs because prescription drugs are the engine of the whole drug industry. Research and sales of prescription drugs are what give the industry its momentum.

The promotion is aimed at doctors because only doctors have the legal right to prescribe, in effect forming a gate through which all prescription drugs must pass. There are critics of the drug industry, including many doctors, who feel that the whole drug prescribing system is overheated with a negative impact on the health of a sizeable portion of the population. But although the health-care system has such critics, their influence must be minimal because drug use and sales, as charted by stock analysts, continue to soar.

Just what are these critics saying? Let us consider in more depth the quality of the gate for drugs – the prescribing doctors. Drugs are not inert substances passing like sand through the body; they interfere in some way with normal body processes, with the potential of doing serious harm as well as conferring some benefit. Doctors are supposed to assess the patient's biology and make a decision about the intended benefits of the drug versus the hazards of taking it. The decision almost always goes in favour of taking a drug; as already noted, it is hard to get out of a doctor's office without a drug prescription.

You would think that, with doctors prescribing what are powerful biological interveners to every patient who walks through the door, they would know a lot about the drugs they prescribe. In fact, most doctors have scant training in the pharmacology of drugs, that is, a scientific understanding of how drugs act within the human body.

Walter Model, a professor of pharmacology at Cornell University Medical Center, New York, teaches pharmacology to medical students; at least, he tries to. He complains that the medical curriculum allows too little time for the subject. The best he could do as a teacher was to say, 'here is a disease and here are one or two drugs you can use to treat the disease.'[5]

Medical students learn very little about how drugs actually intervene in their patients' biology. What they come away with is the belief expressed by D. M. Davies of Durham, England: 'Most present day [medical] students seem to have been born with the firm conviction that medicines can do nothing but good, and ought to be given out at every possible opportunity. Powerful propaganda may sometimes correct this bias but it rarely reverses it.'[6]

Medical students, as mentioned earlier, spend practically all their time learning how to diagnose diseases, the slogan being hammered in by their instructors: 'you can't treat a disease if you don't know what it is.' Disease, once diagnosed, then follows a prescribed course of treatment and the drugs are given automatically. In other words, each disease has a handbook list of drugs. Medical students leave medical school with a shallow knowledge of what drugs do in the human body, and unless they specialize in pharmacology, their knowledge goes no deeper.

Some readers may challenge the contention that learning ceases after medical school. What I am suggesting is that doctors' understanding of the science of impact of drugs on the human body does not deepen. The learning process does indeed go on, but the main driving force in the education of the doctor is now the drug industry. Drug companies spend more on the education of each doctor in practice per year than the doctor ever spent as a student for a year in medical school. The education is obviously biased towards the products the company has to sell, and the companies, like the old song, tend to accentuate the positive and downplay the negative of their products. US drug companies spend as much as 25 per cent of their sales dollars on promotion.

The various drug companies make similar products which compete for each disease, so for every patient visit each company naturally wants the doctor to write a prescription for its product. Promotion of a company's products to doctors has little to do with science, and in fact can be downright frivolous. Joel Lexchin, a Toronto physician concerned about over-use of drugs in medical practice, tells of a drug salesperson who accidentally left a page from his sales manual in a physician's office. The manual gives explicit instructions how to get doctors' attention: hand out cookies in the shape and colour of the company's drug capsules, pizzas with drug initials spelled out in pepperoni, Easter baskets containing eggs painted to represent drug capsules.[7]

Drug company salespersons (also called detailmen) regularly visit doctors' offices and explain the virtues of their companies' products to the doctors. Major drug companies maintain one such salesperson for each 10–20 doctors and this salesperson may visit each doctor on his list some fifty times a year.[8] The drug salesperson promotes the advantages of the drugs and downplays the adverse side-effects. A Finnish study showed, in fact, that the salesperson only mentioned side-effects in one quarter of his visits, and the possibility of alternative therapy on only 10 per cent of the visits. Many doctors feel that the drug salespeople are the easiest way for them to get information about new products and keep up with packaging and dose changes. The doctor gets, in fact, two messages: that a particular disease can be treated only with a drug, and that the product made by the particular company is the best choice.

One purpose of advertising is to keep product names and company names before doctors at all times. Medical journals often contain as many or more pages of glossy, sophisticated advertisements as of original articles, and such advertisements are a major source of income for medical organizations. Although they are sophisticated promoters of products, the advertisements are not necessarily accurate conveyers of medical information. Joe Collier, a clinical pharmacologist at St George's Hospital Medical School, London, gave a graphic illustration. A single issue of the *British Medical Journal* contained twenty-eight full-page advertisements for drugs. Eleven of them, according to Collier, misled doctors by downplaying possible hazards to patients; they were in fact illegal, in breach of the Medicines Act 1968.[9]

When you receive a prescription you presumably believe that the doctor has used the best of medical science and knowledge to prescribe what is in your best interests. How does this presumption square with a 1986 promotion of the Ayerst Laboratories division of American Home Products for its antihypertensive drug, Inderal Long-Acting? Ayerst offered free airline tickets to anywhere in the United States to every doctor who prescribed the drug to fifty patients and filled out a market survey. Ayerst, when criticized for being unethical, defended its action by saying that the prizes included a choice of air travel, diagnostic equipment or medical book. The prize was a 'modest' honorarium for the paperwork.[10]

Another drug company, Squibb Canada, with a competing antihypertensive drug, Capoten, was even more generous than Ayerst; it offered an expensive personal computer to any Canadian doctor who put ten patients on Capoten. Dan Burns, a vice-president of Squibb, said the company retained ownership of the computers, but the doctors could keep them as long as they wanted. He denied that the computer would encourage doctors to prescribe Capoten over another drug. 'I'm trying to be as candid as possible,' he said to a newspaper reporter. 'We don't look at it that way.'[11] Joel Lexchin, a non-believer in the tooth fairy, called the computers a 'very attractive bribe'.

To say that doctors are professional, well trained in the art and science of medicine and therefore resistant to puffed-up claims about drug products is naïve. They are human, and drug advertisers are smart enough to know what works in their promotion. They have convinced most doctors, for example, to prescribe an antiobiotic to all patients with a sore throat.

Anthony Dixon, a family physician in Hamilton, Ontario, once a believer in this piece of conventional wisdom, finally asked himself why he gave an antibiotic to practically every patient who came through the door complaining of a sore throat. He said that 41 per cent of all the prescriptions he had written for the last ten years were for antibiotics. Why? Most sore throats are caused by viruses against which antibiotics are useless. Dixon quoted a study of patients with sore throats in Rhode Island which found that 85 per cent of them were given an antibiotic without the doctor ever finding out whether or not the infection was due to a bacterium. Dixon said that after ten years of routinely prescribing antibiotics for sore throats, he was going to be brave and resist the temptation to prescribe.[12]

Anthony Dixon's conversion is rare. Jerry Avorn, an associate professor of social medicine at Harvard, finds that there is no systematic programme that gives physicians unbiased information about drugs. He and his colleagues did a small-scale experiment in which they counter-detailed 141 doctors with objective information about the effectiveness of drugs in three drug categories. In the nine months following these visits the doctors reduced their prescriptions by 13 per cent. Avorn said that when he went to the government health agencies that paid the drug bills to propose that counter-detailing be expanded, the bureaucrats were not interested.[13]

Back to the Magic Bullet

How important are images in directing science, in this case scientific medicine? Scientists use images or metaphors in their work all the time.

When faced with complex and mysterious phenomena, they use some common everyday event or machine as a symbol to organize their thoughts. Jonathan Miller, in his book *The Body in Question*,[14] comments that we were unable to think of the human heart as a pump until mechanical pumps were in widespread use in the seventeenth century to pump water from mines and through fountains. The idea of blood circulating around the body, pumped by the heart, seems straightforward now, but it is a recent idea in human history. For thousands of years people knew that there was a heart in the chest and that blood flowed from a punctured body. They had only to look at chopped-up victims of battles. But they had no concept that blood flowed all the time in the body. The Roman physician, Galen, in the second century AD likened the heart to a smelter, or furnace, that purified the blood. You could even see the smoke rising from the lungs on a cold day, according to Galen. Smelters purify metals, and Miller says that the smelter was the only image that Galen had available to him.

It was not until some 1,400 years later, in 1628, however, that the English anatomist, William Harvey, applied the pump image to the heart. It gave Harvey the insight he needed to work out the circulation of blood and he was the first to publish the concept that the blood circulates around the body – *pumped* by the heart.

It is not hard to see where the image of the magic bullet comes from. Bullets with their penetrating power are much more surgical than a slashing sword and the myth of magic bullets has been extolled in legend, even becoming the subject of an opera (*Der Freischutz* by C. von Weber). It was the German medical researcher, Paul Ehrlich (1854–1915), who applied the myth to drug science. He suggested that drugs could be invented that like a magic bullet would seek out the diseased tissue and make it whole. If Ehrlich were alive today, he might have used the image of a heat-seeking missile, accurately tracking its hot target.

Ehrlich studied medicine and chemistry at a time when the chemical industry of Germany dominated the world, particularly in the manufacture of synthetic dyes. Ehrlich studied how these dyes coloured body tissues and found that they stained only certain tissues or certain parts of tissues and cells. Ehrlich reasoned that if the dyes, which are synthetic chemicals, sought out and bound to selected tissues, then other chemicals – drugs – could do the same thing. The notion of the magic bullet was born, a drug that would target the diseased tissue and correct the problem.

Ehrlich, a brilliant experimentalist, determined to prove that his idea of the magic bullet worked in human patients. The major medical problems of that era were infectious diseases, and Ehrlich chose to work with one of the more prominent infections, syphilis. To do this kind of research, one needs a laboratory model, and Ehrlich had one in the form of rabbits infected with syphilis. Was it possible to cure the rabbits with a synthetic chemical? Ehrlich had no way of predicting in advance what chemicals, if any, would work, so he tested a shelf-full of chemicals. He had the faith of Columbus who sailed on believing that there was land somewhere in the west. Ehrlich believed that in one of those bottles was the magic bullet for syphilis.

He administered chemical after chemical to his syphilitic rabbits to see if the chemical cured the disease and – importantly – did not kill the rabbits. After 605 failures, his 606th chemical worked. Physicians tried it on human patients and reported miraculous cures. The fact that this chemical did not actually work as well as early reports suggested failed to dampen medical enthusiasm. Chemical number 606, named Salvarsan, became an overnight sensation in the medical world, because it not only showed that a synthetic chemical could treat a deadly infectious disease, it showed that Ehrlich's notion of a magic bullet worked in practice.

Salvarsan was marketed in 1910, and that date could be considered to mark the start of the synthetic drug industry. (It remained on the market for use against syphilis until 1943, when it was supplanted by penicillin.) But in terms of founding a new industry, Salvarsan was a slow start. Not until some twenty-five years later, in 1935, did the industry really blast off with the invention of a class of synthetic drugs, the sulfonamides. Salvarsan is active against one infectious disease, syphilis, but the sulfonamides are effective against a whole spectrum of infecting germs. The discovery of the sulfonamides delivered a message to most of the major chemical companies of the world that synthetic drugs offered a profitable new line of business. Numerous new drug companies sprang up and today, the drug industry sells some $100 billion worth of drugs each year.[15]

The magic bullet idea perpetuates the mechanical image of the human body, the idea that the drug acts exclusively on a defective part of the body. Take a defective brake drum on the family car. Repair the drum, and operation of the car is fully restored. The mechanical problem, the defective brake drum, is treated in an isolated manner: the defect and repair affect no other part, and the garage mechanic can specialize in brake drums. This view of the human body as a machine composed of separate parts directs one's thinking to a specific part, isolated from the rest of the body and – most importantly – isolated from the personal and social environment of the individual. In short, the idea of the magic bullet is one of the most powerful reinforcers of the biomedical model.

How Do Drug Companies Invent New Drugs?

Science has made enormous advances since Ehrlich's day in understanding of the human body and of biology in general, and made great strides in relating the welfare of all species with each other. You might think that this new understanding would render obsolete an old metaphor like that of the magic bullet. But the metaphor is championed by the drug industry. 'What's wrong with that?', stock analysts will say. 'It stimulates the search for new drugs; it's a money-making metaphor.' It is, indeed, difficult to separate how the metaphor is applied to ease the burden of illness from its money-making potential, particularly when we consider the method by which drugs are invented.

Although some drugs have been designed by virtue of knowing in detail some body process, the majority are invented by the method designed by Ehrlich and what crudely might be called the slot machine or fruit machine approach: if you keep pulling the handle often enough you are bound to hit the jackpot.

When Ehrlich discovered Salvarsan he had an experimental model in the form of rabbits with syphilis (his slot machine). He injected the rabbit slot machine with test chemical after test chemical, and finally, on the 606th try, he won. There was no way Ehrlich could have predicted in advance that chemical number 606 was the winner. He had a lot more chemicals than 606 waiting to test, and in fact, if he had by chance picked chemical 606 on his first test, he would have had a winner on his first try.

Drug companies, ninety years later, still employ Ehrlich's two-pronged approach: a chemical and a test system. Chemicals are relatively easy to make; the big hurdle in drug discovery is devising a test system that models some human disease or ailment. Ehrlich had his syphilitic rabbits. In fact, infectious diseases, in general, are easy to model. Disease-causing bacteria and viruses can be grown in test tubes, and many of these organisms infect mice or other laboratory animals.

But there are major categories of human affliction and disease that are difficult to model in the laboratory: for example, cardiovascular disease, mental disorders and pain. Test systems used to model human pain, for example, are only a crude approximation. One such system consists of a rat and a hot plate. The rat's tail is touched to the hot plate and the time the animal takes to flick its tail is recorded. When the rat is given an experimental painkiller drug, flick time is slower. The rat presumably is less bothered by the smoking tail.

A typical large company employs several hundred chemists who synthesize new chemicals. The advantage of having your own chemists is that the chemicals they synthesize can be patented. Each new chemical is tested (screened) in a battery of fifty-odd test systems. The company hopes that a candidate chemical will show a positive action in one or more of their laboratory test systems. The chances are that the chemical will show negative in all fifty test systems. But since a company may be testing 200 or more chemicals a week, it will find several that are active in one or more tests.

But a candidate chemical active in a test system is far from being a commercial drug. This is only the start. The company has to think ahead to where it can make the most money. Although the company may have fifty different test systems, it puts special emphasis into those areas with big commerical payoffs. The big money-making areas are relatively few: heart, bacterial infections (real or imagined), ulcers, anxiety and pain. Two of these categories, heart and infections, alone account for 28 per cent of all drug sales.[16] Drug companies bias development of new drugs to the big sales categories. Their screening of new chemicals may indeed turn up candidate drugs for other less profitable categories, but unless the company is able to forecast adequate sales, the drug remains on the shelf.

Having discovered a chemical that shows positive action in one of their big sales categories, the drug company must undertake long and tedious testing to see how toxic it is. Such testing takes five to seven years, and most candidate drugs, even though they show good activity in the test system, are knocked out because they are toxic in some way.

In any event, the slot machine process eventually turns up a winning drug in one of the favoured categories and this is licensed for sale by the government. Hoffman–La Roche, a drug company that concentrates on vitamins, sedatives and antidepressants (Vitamin C, Valium, Librium), says that it has to test 10,000 chemicals before finding one that can be marketed.[17] Although such research seems chancy and expensive – $50–100 million per single new drug – the large drug companies have the resources to test enough new chemicals each year so that, by the law of the slot machine, they hit the jackpot eventually. Payoffs are elephantine. SmithKline Beckman Corporation, Philadelphia,[18] is reported to have spent $50 million developing its new anti-ulcer drug, Tagamet. The company estimated that it would sell $400 million worth of this drug a year. It was wrong: Tagamet sales in its third year on the market (1987) hit one billion dollars.

You read about the success of the industry in the financial journals. *Fortune* Magazine called the Merck Company, Rahway, NJ, America's most admired firm. Merck is admired, not because it makes and sells 100 different prescription drugs, but because it made 34 per cent profit on its $5.1 billion sales in 1987 and moreover has the means to keep rolling up those profits. It has one of the best research laboratories in the industry with fifty new drugs moving through its development pipeline to be marketed shortly. It is enough to excite the most jaded stockbroker.

The drug industry as a whole is considered one of the most lucrative sectors in the financial community. This community, in particular, applauds the big winner, and the real big winners in the view of stock specialists are drugs that top one billion dollars in annual sales.

In 1988, four drugs hit this stratospheric target: two for treating ulcers and two for lowering blood pressure. The two anti-ulcer drugs are Tagamet, made by SmithKline Beckman, and Zantac, made by Glaxo Holdings, a British company. The blood pressure drugs are Vasotec, one of Merck's 100 products, and Capoten of computer fame, made by Squibb.

These billion-dollar drugs offer companies exceptional opportunity to grow, according to Neal Sweig, a security analyst for Prudential–Bache: 'Most of the giant drug companies of today became giants from having a very successful drug or two or three.'[19] Obviously every small drug company hopes it will be catapulted into the winner's circle by hitting a drug jackpot. And the ones already there know they have to keep running to stay on top. Roy Vagelos, Merck's chairman, has said, 'you'll die if you sit on your laurels.'[20] So all the companies keep looking for more big winners.

This search for the big sales winner skews drug research, as already noted, into a few product categories. Both ulcers and high blood pressure, which are symptoms of deeper problems, can be corrected in most instances by non-drug means, but that fact is not going to excite the stock market. The fact is that the preferred treatment of all manner of human illness is drug technology, and although it is based on a scientific metaphor (the magic bullet), this technology above all is a commercial venture, driven by the forces of the financial markets.

The Biomedical Model Can Distort Social Policy

The biomedical model (which includes the magic bullet image) is not without its critics. One such, Allan Brandt, professor of social medicine and health policy at Harvard University, comments that while the mechanical aspects of the biomedical model have their place – the model has been a powerful intellectual force in the development of useful drugs and treatment – that is not enough. Speaking of infectious diseases, Brandt says that it is not enough to think of the problem as an infecting parasite and a person infected; you have to see the problem in terms of all the connections between parasite, infected person and all the social and environmental forces. And, he drives the point home: all these relations are fluid, ever changing; a static, mechanical model of health and disease is unable to accommodate the changing scene.[21] Brandt notes that neither Ehrlich's Salvarsan nor pencillin solved the problem of syphilis. Both drugs at first offered some control of the disease, but the syphilis parasite became resistant to the drugs and social habits changed. The disease is not going away. In fact, the American Centers for Disease Control in 1987 reported a 30 per cent increase in the incidence of syphilis in the United States.

Critics like Brandt call for an enlarged perspective of health and disease; but the biomedical model is the arrangement of stars chosen by medical practice as its navigational guide. It is important to understand how static that arrangement is, and in particular, how it can distort social policy when dealing with the fluid, complex processes of all stages of life.

Consider ageing: a natural process that has come to be highly distorted by over-dependence on drugs. The older a person becomes, the more drugs are prescribed. Each resident of the Province of Ontario aged 65 years or over consumes at least 30 prescriptions a year and the provincial department of health, which pays for these drugs, finds with alarm that some seniors consume over 200 prescriptions a year. The Ontario Minister of Health, Elinor Caplan, believes that Ontarians – not just the seniors – are the most highly medicated people on earth.[22] Caplan has no idea of what to do about it, though, because she is reluctant to interfere with a doctor's right to prescribe and a patient's right to be drugged. Moreover, the drugging is not always beneficial: the Royal College of Physicians, London, found that 10 per cent of all elderly patients admitted to hospital were admitted because of adverse drug reactions.[23]

Do drugs solve the social problem of how to manage an ageing population? Daniel Callahan, director of the Hastings Center, a public policy organization, notes that the mechanical view of the human body invites doctors to use every advance in drugs and machines to extend an elderly person's life for another few months. 'A cruel imbalance,' he says, 'exists between support for life-extending, high-technology medicine and that less fancy medicine necessary for a decent quality of life, notably affordable, long-term institutional care and decent home care.'[24]

Thomas McKeown, professor of social medicine at the University of Birmingham, England, is another critic who believes we should pay more attention to the natural rhythms of life. He points out that a baby, having survived the ruthless selection of conception and the fetal stage, should have the potential to lead a robust, disease-free life.[25] The social reality, he finds, is the reverse; people and their health-care institutions believe that the human body is prone to breakdown and that only the heroic ministering of high-technology medicine (with heavy emphasis on drugs) pulls people through life. In studying the basis for human health McKeown concluded that in fact social and environmental factors play the major role in determining the level of health in populations; the health-care system and its drugs play only a marginal role.

The views of Callahan and McKeown fall outside the conventional wisdom as attested by the buoyant market in drug company stock. But I do not believe that either critic would do away with high medical technology. The issue, as Callahan notes, is not that drug technology is intrinsically bad but that the health-care system seems incapable of promoting alternatives. And among those alternatives is greater acknowledgement of the role the natural environment plays in maintaining the health of the population.

4

The One-basket Health Policy

What drives the health-care system of industrialized countries? Is it the medical doctors, the government health bureaucracies, people's desire for good health? They all do in a sense, but the main engine that propels the health-care system is high medical technology and the industries that develop and sell the technology. The drug industry, of course, is very much part of this high-technology sector and, as we noted previously, it has become a force in the lives of consumers, the majority of whom consume its products daily. But medical technology also includes medical equipment, diagnostic services, hospitals; and medical care revolves around this technology. Medical care, in fact, could be said to be application of this technology to consumers, who in their ready acceptance of it have come to equate their health with machines, drugs and laboratory tests. This almost total reliance for health care on high medical technology is paradoxical, because in spite of its power to manipulate human biology, this technology fails to deliver on much of its promise of health. It is indeed a tribute to the almost universal acceptance of the technology that its failures are all but ignored.

The grip of high medical technology on the health-care system has its drawbacks, one of which is that alternative approaches to health that are equal to or better than high medical technology – and much cheaper – tend to be ignored or suppressed. One is unlikely to find any drive for environmental protection coming from the providers of high medical technology. Thus our goal of understanding why the health-care system fails to provide any insight into the connection between health and the environment leads us to look more closely at the leverage exerted by high medical technology on health policy.

This chapter takes up two issues, one hotly debated in public fora, the other barely rating a mention. Health policy is of course a hot topic among politicians, but although they may talk about improving the public's health, their way of improving health centres on making high medical technology accessible to everyone. The debate swirls around how to make accessibility more efficient and how to cap costs. The basic assumption of the debaters is that accessibility ensures health.

The second issue, the quiet issue that receives little attention among politicians and analysts of health policy, is lack of systematic examination of whether or not specific procedures – operations, medical treatments – are effective. How do we know that having a particular operation or taking a drug, on average, makes patients healthier than they would be without that operation or drug? I touched on this point earlier when discussing drugs: antibiotics, for example, although powerful interveners in one's biology, are given freely for sore throats when in about 80 per cent of cases the drug contributes nothing and indeed may be harmful.

Not only is there lack of evaluation of individual medical procedures, there is lack of effort to evaluate systematically the contribution of the whole expensive system of high medical technology to the health of the population. Overall, is the health of the public best served by the one-basket, high-tech approach to health?

The Medical–Industrial Complex

High medical technology by itself is neutral. It is not the technology *per se* that makes health policy good or bad: it is the institutions that use it. So this chapter is not to be taken as a critique of high medical technology, but a critique of its use and misuse.

The one institution that gives high medical technology its life and direction lacks a formal name but is often referred to as the *medical–industrial complex*, a group of industries that develops and markets drugs, medical equipment and supplies and provides a variety of health services. It is closely bound up with the medical profession – absolutely essential for the industry – because only physicians can legally apply medical technology and services to patients. In other words, the industry can only market its products and services through medical doctors. The companies make their money selling their goods and services, the physicians make their money applying the technology; hence the tightness of the complex.

The medical–industrial complex is no small industry. It employs some 10 million people in the United States and comparable numbers in other countries. It operates just as effectively in countries like Britain and Sweden with government-run health-care systems, because these systems are equally dependent on the technologies and services of the medical–industrial complex. It is in the United States, however, that the complex perhaps receives most attention and that public argument over its role in health care is most abrasive. But it is hard to detect in that argument any interest in a place for a preventive health strategy. Rather, public argument revolves around the efficiency of the complex – does it cost too much for the health care it delivers?

The term 'medical–industrial complex' is not a term the industry itself uses; the term is not intended to be laudatory. It derives from President Eisenhower's warning of thirty years ago against the growing and insidious influence of the military–industrial complex. Eisenhower in the last days of his presidency warned that the influence of this complex would distort military and social policy by virtue of its heavy bias towards the manufacture of the hardware of warfare. He saw military policy being dictated by the needs of the defence industry rather than by the defence needs of the country.

Some doctors have the same thought in mind. They dislike being handmaidens to the medical–industrial complex with its million-dollar machines and services, which they say overwhelms health policy and distorts the practice of medicine.

How do doctors define the medical–industrial complex? One doctor, Stanley Wohl, a specialist in internal medicine at the Stanford University Medical Center, defines the complex as a group of companies that make medically related machines and drugs and sell health services.[1] Wohl's list of companies is populated by such names as American Hospital Supply, Beecham Services, IBM, McDonnell Douglas, Dow Chemical, American Cyanamid, Hoffmann–La Roche, Humana, and so on. These corporations take in one third of every dollar spent in the United States on health care (some $200 billion out of a total expenditure of $600 billion in 1989). This huge proportion of total receipts is concentrated in a relatively small number of large corporations whose influence on delivery of health care is governed, according to Wohl, by the rule of the stock market. Short-term gain, financial growth and the bottom line all count for more than the patient's best interests. Wohl is not against high-tech medicine, but he sees the control of that technology passing from physicians to hospital and corporate accountants. He notes that physicians have always been subject to a central conflict between self-interest and altruism but feels that any hope of altruism is lost when decision-making passes to persons 'whose main concern is efficient administration and cost containment'.[2]

What Wohl is really talking about is power. Who controls the delivery of health care, the doctors or the administrators of the medical–industrial complex? Let us put this question in even more fundamental terms. As mentioned in previous chapters, doctors, by virtue of their medical school training, uphold a conceptual model under which they practise medicine – the biomedical model. This model embraces one-cause/one-effect thinking: that is, diagnosis reveals a cause of the disease and getting at the cause relieves the effect – the disease. Normally this concept of a human ill and what to do about it would be subject to constant buffeting and reshaping by new ideas within universities and professional organizations. And over time, the model and the underlying approach to the public's health could be expected to evolve in a more open direction. But in Wohl's view, control over evolution of the biomedical model has shifted to the medical–industrial complex; and this complex has a vested interest in hanging on to the cause-and-effect rules of the biomedical model because they justify the complex's equipment and services.

From its controlling position the medical–industrial complex sets the rules for playing the health-care game. The situation is akin to the game of American football, in which professional players have invested years in honing their talents, and the public has long been conditioned to expect the game to be played in a certain way. Imagine the outcry from the players, the equipment manufacturers and the public if they were told that American-style football is out and the players have to play European-style football (soccer) and the fans are going to have to learn the finer points of this new (to them) game. It is not likely to happen. In the same way, any shift in the rules of the biomedical model, for example, towards prevention is unlikely, because it would jeopardize the investment and way of doing business of the medical–industrial complex.

The barrier to thinking about ways to improve public health imposed by the medical–industrial complex alarms those critics who see the public's health in its broader social context, who recognize that there is more to health than machines and high-tech services. Thomas Lambo, Deputy Director-General of the World Health Organization (WHO), is one official who notes the waning interest among government policy-makers in alternative approaches to public health. Lambo observes that since the 1970s the world health picture is falling apart. Health, he says, cannot be considered a problem for doctors and health workers alone: 'There are too many variables.' Lambo cites poverty and politics as the reasons for a worldwide decline in health.[3]

Joseph Califano, Jr, is another official who knows the politics of which Lambo speaks. He was Secretary of Health Education and Welfare of the United States, 1977–9, and in a book about the American health scene, he writes of the unhealthy 'domination of the political power by the health-care providers [his term for the medical–industrial complex].'[4] The domination is obviously highly successful because, as Califano notes, the cost of health care extracted by the providers is rising at twice the rate of inflation, thanks to government handouts and a generous policy towards those providers. The United States spends as much on health care as on the military and education combined, almost 12 per cent of the Gross National Product. By the year 2000 the proportion of the nation's wealth devoted to high-tech medical care is expected to reach 15 per cent.

You can see the power of the medical–industrial complex to extract money from citizens' pockets in the way hospitals operate. They have become the fortresses of the health-care system, and certainly they are where the full technological force of the medical–industrial complex is brought to bear. *Harpers Magazine* describes the force applied to one patient, Mary K., in the intensive care unit of a New York city hospital.[5] The hospital staff performed an average of twenty-six technical procedures on Mary K. each day of her stay, from a blood count costing $17.00 to the monitoring of blood gases on a machine rented for $354 a day. Her hospital bed cost a mere $500 a day; her twenty-six procedures cost $1,973.10 a day, four times as much, and these charges did not include her doctors' costs. Mary K.'s bills ended with her death three and a half weeks after admission. Mary K. apparently had a fatal disease that no amount of high technology could reverse. This did not deter the hospital staff from poking, injecting, sampling Mary K.'s body two dozen times a day while she lay dying.

It is this seemingly unnecessary – and expensive – activity that galls some politicians, like Representative Patricia Schroeder of the US Congress. 'When you look at the Federal dollar and how it's spent on medical care,' she said, 'a very high percentage of it is spent on the last few days of someone's life.'[6] Schroeder made her comment to emphasize the unevenness of how health dollars are spent; there seem to be few available for low-tech health care at all stages of life.

But the bottom line for the medical–industrial complex is that although critics like Lambo, Califano and Schroeder are trying to tone down what they consider the excessive use of high medical technology and divert resources to alternatives, their views are not diverting health policy-makers from providing more high-tech medicine. It is hard for politicians to resist what John O'Brien-Bell, president of the Canadian Medical Association, says is the duty of doctors. He was quoted as saying that doctors have a duty to lobby governments for the latest medical equipment, partly because if they do not give their patients the most advanced treatment they (the doctors) are subject to lawsuits.[7]

O'Brien-Bell's comment is an acknowledgement of the fact that both doctors and their patients subscribe to what Aaron Wildavsky, of the Graduate School of Public Policy, University of California, calls the Great Medical Equation: medical care = health.[8] But this is a false equation, according to Wildavsky: 'The best estimates are that the medical system (doctors, drugs, hospitals) affects about 10 percent of the usual indices for measuring health.'

In other words, 90 per cent of all illness is unaffected by high-tech medicine; most illness is self-limiting. Either the individual gets better anyway, or the illness is fatal and no amount of medicine prevents the outcome. This is not to say that medical care cannot ease symptoms or suffering, or slow down a fatal illness; just that much of it is applied in an inappropriate way and options for less expensive and equally effective care are not provided by the health-care system.

Medicare in the United States

While saying it is the duty of doctors to lobby for more high-tech equipment, O'Brien-Bell also said that it is up to the government to decide what society needs. The statement is self-serving because it relieves doctors of any requirement to be more judicious in their use of high medical technology, putting the onus on governments. But politicians tend to reflect what they perceive the public wants, and when it comes to health they interpret the public's desire for good health as a desire for access to the latest and most elaborate medical procedures. And indeed, health policy in the industrialized nations for the past several decades has concentrated almost exclusively on making high medical technology accessible to everyone.

To explore this point further, we will look at two government health programmes: Medicare in the United States and the National Health Service in Britain.

First Medicare. The United States lacks a single, universal health programme comparable to the government health services of Sweden and Britain. There is a mosaic of programmes in the American health sector, but the thrust of all of them is the same – access to high-tech medical care. The method of paying for that access, however, varies, with a mixture of private and government payment. And surprisingly, although the United States is thought of as the ultimate in free-market medicine, the federal government finances 40 per cent of the country's medical bills. Medicare is the centrepiece of these programmes, providing medical cover to 33 million Americans who are disabled or 65 years of age and older. As the following anecdote suggests, this cover is not without its glitches.

In October 1987, Helen Bennett, 72, of Massapequa, New York, was diagnosed as having a tumour in her chest. Her long-time doctor, Arthur Berken, wanted to put her in hospital for chemotherapy, but Mrs Bennett, living alone, did not want to leave her dog, so she asked if she could have the course of treatments in Berken's office. He agreed, and over the next three weeks, Mrs Bennett spent two hours a day, four times a week, receiving the anti-cancer drugs Adriamycin and Dacarbazine.

But the system of Medicare disbursement has become highly bureaucratic and expensive to administer, and moreover, it tries to direct treatment without regard to cost or benefit to patient. Thus, although Mrs Bennett's treatment proceeded to the satisfaction of both patient and doctor, the trouble began when Dr Berken tried to bill the Medicare plan. According to the *New York Times*, which reported the situation, Berken received an anonymous computer printout saying that his treatment 'was not reasonable and necessary'.[9] How could Medicare make a value judgement without any knowledge of what's going on? Berken asked. He explained that chemotherapy is generally given in hospital, but Mrs Bennett being an outpatient could go home every day, a cheaper arrangement than spending three weeks in hospital. He tried phoning the Medicare office but received more unsigned printouts rejecting the claim. Exasperated, Berken contacted his Congressman, Robert Mrazek, and solicited his help in finding 'one human being to explain to me their logic'.

Mrazek, who presumably would rather be dealing with national affairs, was so overloaded with similar Medicare complaints from his constituents – 240 in the past year – that he hired a full-time assistant to help sort out the problems. In the case of Helen Bennett, it was several months before Berken, Mrazek's assistant and a *New York Times* reporter managed to track down the 'one human being' they were after: Gloria McCarthy, of a private insurance company contracted by the government to handle Medicare claims, Empire Bluecross–Blue Shield. McCarthy, head of the company's Medicare outpatient programme, said that Empire Bluecross was reconsidering its outpatient chemotherapy policy and that most such claims would now be paid. But until Berken, and apparently other doctors, complained, the Medicare insurance company tried to force patients into the more expensive hospitals by witholding payment for outpatient care.

To understand why Dr Berken had difficulty in recovering his outpatient fee is to understand one reason for the ballooning cost of Medicare. When the Medicare bill was signed into law by President Johnson in 1965, it was thought the cost to the government would be modest. In 1967 the programme cost only $3.4 billion, but by 1987, that cost had risen to $158 billion and was still rising. Joseph Califano predicts that this one government programme alone will cost American taxpayers $600 billion by the year 2000.

As long ago as 1936, the federal government wanted to attach a health-care plan to social security legislation, but opposition from organized medicine, namely the American Medical Association (AMA), so cowed Congressmen that the idea of health benefits for the elderly was dropped. The AMA's lobbying against such legislation continued, and when the idea of a Medicare programme was resurrected in the 1960s, Congressmen realized that the programme would not work without the doctors' co-operation. Congress made substantial concessions to both doctors and hospitals in order to get the legislation passed, concessions that are at the root of Medicare's problems today.

AMA's main opposition to Medicare, which it called socialized medicine, was that it did not want any party coming between doctor and patient. The doctors wanted no interference in how they practised medicine or billed patients. But by the mid-1960s doctors were accustomed to private insurance plans that paid a fee to the doctor or hospital for each patient and for each service rendered. The major insurance carriers in this area were Blue Cross for doctors' bills and Blue Shield for hospital bills, and both carriers were structured to serve the interests of doctors and hospitals. The government, in passing the Medicare legislation, agreed that it would simply foot the bill and that administration of Medicare would be handled through the private insurance carriers. Doctors like Berken simply bill the regional insurance company administering Medicare.

Paul Starr, a Harvard sociologist who has studied the evolution of the American health-care system, noted that in this act, 'the federal government surrendered direct control of the programme and its costs.'[10] In fact, it not only surrendered control over costs, it surrendered control over the introduction and use of high-tech medicine, one reason why in the United States evaluation of new medical technology is virtually non-existent. The medical–industrial complex can develop a piece of equipment or a new procedure and introduce it into wide use – paid for by Medicare or other insurance programmes – unhampered by awkward questions about whether or not it benefits people's health.

Although American politicians do not argue about the bills of individual patients (Helen Bennett's chemotherapy treatments cost $17,000), they do argue over the free flight of the overall bill for Medicare. There is an unending argument between politicians and the medical–industrial complex over how to control costs. But the one question politicians do not seem to ask is whether or not all this medical service is necessary. It is not a question of politicians seemed inclined to raise, because they believe their constituents want the service and that it is the politicians' duty to ensure that people have access to it. Yet the accelerating costs are driving more critics to question the need for so much medical attention. Robert Evans, a Canadian health economist, says the argument that people need the level of health care provided by such government programmes as Medicare is 'advanced only in ignorance or deliberate deception'.[11]

One reason consumers demand all these medical services, Evans notes, is that they are poorly informed about the contribution of these services to their health and, therefore, rely on the judgement of doctors, who make money every time they provide a service. But it is not just the consumers who are poorly informed; as I have already mentioned, the doctors themselves often have only a rudimentary idea of the effectiveness of the procedures they employ. Few medical procedures have been objectively evaluated for their ability to improve the patient's health. More seriously, the overall health outcome of Medicare itself has never been examined. Is this the best way for the country to spend its health dollars?

Babies Fall through the Cracks: A Commentary on Medicare

The difference in cost and health returns between high-tech and low-tech medical care can be illustrated by a look at the start of the age spectrum. The US National Commission to Prevent Infant Mortality says that every year 40,000 American babies born to poor mothers fail to reach their first birthday, many because they are small and born too soon from lack of pre-natal care. (It has been estimated that 600,000 pregnant women in the USA in 1988, poor or not, had little or no pre-natal care.) Pre-natal care and advice that will effectively prevent low birth-weight can be given to each mother for about $400. This is not the kind of service that interests the medical–industrial complex because it is not high-tech and there is not much profit to be made. The

Commission estimates that a low-birth-weight baby, because of its disabilities, can run up lifetime medical costs of over $400,000.[12] And more seriously, from the point of view of the afflicted human, all the high-tech medical services will fail to cure or correct the initial damage suffered in the womb.

It should be mentioned that the USA's 22 million poor are covered by an adjunct programme to Medicare – Medicaid. So medical care is accessible, but one has to ask whether or not government health programmes such as Medicare and Medicaid ensure access to health. They provide access to high-tech medicine, but, as we see, something low-tech like pre-natal care falls through the cracks. The system has become so gigantic and so expensive that public debate centres mostly on how to manage costs without ever examining what the system is delivering – or, more importantly, what the system is not delivering. Joseph Califano notes the discrepancy: 'Of the $550 billion [1988] Americans spend on health care,' he says, 'less than 0.3 per cent is spent on health promotion and disease prevention.'[13]

The British National Health Service

Is the dominance of health care by the medical–industrial complex a phenomenon only of the freewheeling open market of the United States or is it more widespread? Let us look at the British National Health Service, a system of universal health care tightly run by the government.

British politicians, like their American counterparts, worry about the escalating costs of medical care, but the British government, unlike the US, does something about it. Its policy can be seen through the eyes of a hospital administrator, Barrie Dowdeswell, of the Royal Victorian Infirmary in Newcastle.

In 1988, Dowdeswell enlarged the hospital's florist shop and added other profit-making centres in order to swell the hospital's income. He also approached a local Nissan car factory with an offer to run a private health-care facility for employees. Dowdeswell said he would be able to offer the service more cheaply than a private company. Does this sound like a state-run hospital? These entrepreneurial activities are Dowdeswell's response to a firm cap on the budget the government allots to his hospital. Ward beds have already been eliminated – without cutting service, he say – but the fat is cut and the hospital will just have to generate income in other ways. 'If we don't do something ourselves, we condemn this hospital to waiting for a government bailout,' he said in interview. 'And, you won't find much confidence around here of that happening.'[14] In the meantime, the waiting time at the Royal Victorian Infirmary for a patient scheduled for cataract surgery has doubled to one year. Emergency operations to repair aneurysms – a life-threatening condition – had to be postponed several times because of a shortage of skilled nurses.

Dowdeswell and his hospital are caught in a squeeze between the rising costs of high-tech medicine and a government determined to hold costs steady. The British government has for several years held the total cost of its National Health Service at 6.2 per cent of GNP, compared with 9 per cent in Sweden, another country with a national health service. Whereas politicians in the United States dither over the costs of Medicare, the British government simply says no. It can do that because of its highly centralized health-care system. Eighty-six per cent of Britain's health expenditure is paid through the National Health Service; the remainder is paid directly by patients or through private insurance plans.

The National Health Service is also structured in a way that makes it easier to contain costs. It has a two-tier system of doctors. Thirty-five per cent of British doctors practise as independent contractors, called general practitioners (GPs), that is, they are prepared to look after all members of the family. They are the equivalent of family doctors in the United States. General practitioners work in a private office or a community clinic, and each signs up a panel of patients which he or she contracts to look after. Patients select a doctor within their area, establishing a doctor–patient bond – a bond that, ironically, many United States physicians practising in corporate-run clinics have lost. Doctors are paid a capitation fee, a sum for each patient on the panel, regardless of the number of times the patient sees the doctor. A GP has on average 2,200 individuals on his panel, and in the course of a year sees 600 of them with coughs and colds, 325 with skin disorders including dandruff, 100 with chronic rheumatism, 50 with high blood pressure, 8 with heart attacks, 5 with appendicitis and 5 with strokes.[15]

The tier of GPs acts as a primary screen for the National Health Service. GPs treat patients with minor complaints or, if they judge the complaints to be more serious, they refer patients to specialists, called consultants. Consultants occupy the second tier, the top position of privilege and power in the Service. Consultants are attached to a hospital and are relatively few in number. Only about 20 per cent of registered doctors in Britain are consultants, compared with 85 per cent of doctors in the United States who practise a speciality. The National Health Service pays each consultant a salary, and in addition, consultants are allowed a percentage of time to engage in private practice on a fee-for-service basis. Consultants control their own professional standards and have a major voice in the organization and the standard of medical care delivered in their hospitals. Because of their prestige and status, they influence strongly the way the British public and government think about human health.

The work of the consultants revolves around the expensive high-tech medical care delivered by hospitals. In fact, the whole National Health Service revolves around the hospitals and about 65 per cent of the country's doctors (including the consultants) work in hospitals. This is the style of medicine determined by the machines and drugs of the medical–industrial complex. There are differences in degree between British hospitals and American ones, but the high-tech styles are identical. British hospitals tend to have fewer pieces of expensive equipment and because the number of consultant positions in each hospital is controlled, they have, for example, only half as many surgeons per capita as the United States. British doctors are less inclined to subject their patients to major operations and other high-tech procedures. A heart bypass operation, for instance, is performed about one quarter as often as in the United States, and there seems to be no difference in outcome of patients with heart conditions. In fact, according to Roger Hollingsworth, a sociology professor at the University of Wisconsin, who has compared the medical systems of Britain and the United States, there is no real difference in the level of care.

British doctors may use high technology to a lesser degree, but this does not suggest less faith in the technology. They are just as strong proponents of new and improved technology as their American counterparts. They use expensive high technology less because the equipment is not so readily available. But less expensive technology, such as drugs, they prescribe as freely or even more freely than doctors in the United States.[17]

Although both US and British doctors tend to be paternalistic towards their patients – 'doctor knows best' – British doctors carry paternalism to a far greater extent. The plus side, at least from the point of view of cost containment, is that the British doctor is better able to persuade a patient not to undergo treatments for which there is no benefit. They are able to say, 'look, this is all we can do for your cancer or for your chronic arthritis' – and the patient accepts the decision. Contrast this attitude with that in the United States where treatment ends only with the patient's last breath. A British doctor who worked in an American hospital was astounded at the amount of treatment given patients: 'Rarely does an American doctor state that there is no surgery that would help, no drug that is advantageous, and no further investigation is required. There seems to be an irresistible urge always to do something, even though in many cases the doctor concerned must realize that there is no possibility of benefit.'[18]

The more authoritarian relationship between British doctor and patient has its disadvantages. Arrogance and a faith in the infallibility of their own judgement, means that there is little likelihood of doctors questioning their own belief system of health and disease and even less of admitting that there are alternative ways of preserving health. You can see this arrogance expressed in the fate of one experiment in alternative medical care.

This experiement, set up in the London suburb of Peckham in the 1930s by two medical doctors, Scott Williamson and Innes Pearse, created a total health plan for some 2,000 families. The plan, with its own large social centre, encouraged fitness, social conviviality and good health practices. Williamson, Pearse and their medical staff got to know their families very well, giving them the kind of health maintenance that avoided illness. The plan enjoyed great success for about ten years before it was scrapped in 1948 by the newly introduced National Health Service. There were to be no funds for this type of programme.

A dogged group of British doctors and associates, some of whom once worked in the Peckham programme, have tried to rekindle a similar programme since 1948, but the idea of a wellness programme has been consistently rebuffed both by the British medical societies and by the government health bureaucracy. The belief that prevailed in 1948, that such programmes are unnecessary for health maintenance, prevails still.

The National Health Service was founded on the egalitarian principle that although most people do not mind seeing someone else drive a Rolls-Royce, everyone is entitled to a heart bypass operation. Aneurin Bevan, the minister in the British Labour government responsible for introducing the National Health Service in 1948, firmly believed that when the less advantaged citizens – those then unable to afford health care – had access to doctors and drugs, their diseases would vanish. He predicted that the need for medical facilities would decline. What he did not anticipate was the capacity of the modern health-care system to generate new demand based, in large part, on the patient's desire for access to heart transplants and CT scans. Bevan also made the mistake of equating access to doctors and their technology with access to health.

Bevan did not then, nor does the British government now, see human health in its whole relation to society and the natural environment in the way that Williamson and Pearse did. The government is satisfied to limit its focus on health to gritty debates over hospital budgets and the way the National Health Service is run. A comprehensive legislative approach to human health is just as absent as it is in the United States.

But now, forty years after the introduction of the National Health Service, slogan and fiscal reality clash: costs and demands for expensive medical technology keep pushing on the government's limits. Its response was to restrict hospital services, forcing Barrie Dowdeswell and other hospital managers to ration the services they offer. But now the government has gone further. It announced plans in 1989 to revolutionize the National Health Service, bringing it closer to the American free-market health-care system. 'For the first time since the NHS was founded in 1948, doctors will be encouraged to see patients as revenue sources and expense centres,' said Gordon Best, director of the King's Fund College, an organization that trains health managers.[19]

So it seems the revolution in health care has more to do with management and costs than with health; the obvious intent is to continue universal access to high-tech medical care, but to make it more revenue-effective. British health policy-makers seem no more interested than their American counterparts in questioning Wildavsky's Great Medical Equation that medical care equals health.

Evaluation of Medical Procedures

One of the issues that keeps surfacing is the lack of evaluation of the benefits high-tech medicine confers on its consumers. The issue is important to the central theme of this book because one has to ask why society has elected to put so much of its health resources into high-tech 'cures'. One result is that prevention, like low birth-weight babies, falls through the cracks. The underlying assumption in raising this question is that if we had more objective evidence of just how well high-tech medicine works (or doesn't) it would be easier to assign it a more balanced role in preserving the nation's health. Politicians and society as a whole would be more willing to put resources into prevention, including environmental protection.

The fact that evaluation takes place, however, does not necessarily mean anything changes, if policy-makers are unreceptive. It does not take much to understand the social implications of the low-birth-weight babies. The figures on this issue mentioned previously have been widely known for a long time but, according to statistics of the United States Public Health Service, the percentage of low-birth-weight babies continues to rise.

So, recognizing that trying to change public policy is like trying to change the direction of a glacier, I end the chapter with two accounts which give us some insight into the question of whether or not the value to health of high medical technology is overrated. The first is an evaluation of a specific medical procedure, the heart bypass operation. The second is an evaluation of the whole health-care system.

The Heart Bypass Operation

The beginnings of an ailing heart can actually occur early in life, before puberty. Fatty deposits called plaques start building up in the coronary arteries at an early age in a disease called atherosclerosis. The coronary arteries, which weave through the heart muscle delivering fresh blood with oxygen and fuel, seem particularly vulnerable to this disease. The plaques build up slowly and, like rust in a pipe, they restrict the flow of blood. Eventually, when the plaques block 50 per cent or more of the cross-section of an artery – the individual by now is usually in the fifties or sixties – blood flow may be insufficient to supply enough oxygen during exertion. Climbing stairs may be enough to overload the heart muscle, and, at this point, like a car engine starved of fuel, it sputters under the stress. The result: heart pains known as angina. There are two ways of treating angina – medication combined with dietary and lifestyle changes, or bypass surgery.

The surgery is no simple undertaking. The surgeons hook the patient to a heart and lung machine that routes the blood through a series of exchangers that remove carbon dioxide and infuse oxygen. The development of this machine, which can support a patient long enough for an operation, was the key breakthrough in open heart surgery, enabling the surgeons to cut into the chest and work on a motionless heart. Taking a vein from the patient's leg, surgeons graft it above and below the blockage in a coronary artery, so that it forms a detour or bypass. They may graft three or four such veins, which now take over the task of supplying a section of the heart muscle with blood. Because the new artery is the patient's own flesh, there is no problem with rejection. Patients generally are able to take exercise after the operation without experiencing angina, but would they have done just as well or better with the less traumatic medicine and lifestyle approach?

The coronary artery bypass operation was introduced about twenty years ago and has proved to be enormously popular with surgeons and patients: over 230,000 operations were performed in the United States in 1987, a 50 per cent increase over 1982.[20] This popularity has continued in spite of questions raised about the operation's efficacy, starting with reports in the 1970s that suggested the operation was of only marginal value for some patients. The problem for the patient is that plugged coronary arteries are only symptoms of the basic disease, atherosclerosis. Arterial deterioration is not corrected by the operation, and the plaques continue their relentless buildup. An editorial in the British medical journal, *The Lancet*, noted that 20 per cent of new bypass arteries become plugged within a year. Pain in most patients is relieved at first but returns within a few years.[21]

The alternative treatment to the bypass operation is a combination of drugs, dietary changes and exercise. Reports now coming in suggest that the lifestyle changes can arrest the disease process and may even reverse it. In any event, such treatment is relatively inexpensive and requires no traumatic opening of the chest. A comparison of the respective benefits to patients of the two treatments was the subject of three studies over the last ten years. Two studies done in the United States conclude that there is no difference in longevity of the patients of the two groups, but the third, a European study, suggests that there may be some lengthening of life for patients receiving the bypass operation.

This is the usual state of affairs in science: no clear answer. But heart patients are not uniform, and an editorial in the *New England Journal of Medicine*, commenting on the situation, said that for a small group of seriously diseased patients, the operation can bring about improvement.[22] For the rest of the patients with atherosclerosis, all that is needed is drug therapy, exercise and improved nutrition.

This information has not slowed the demand for the operation in the United States, which continues at four times the rate in Europe, at a cost of $30,000 each. A large number of surgical teams and hospital facilities would become redundant if this enterprise, now worth $6 billion a year in the US, were to slacken in momentum.

The demand continues, because, according to David Feeny and colleagues of McMaster University Medical School, who study the effectiveness of medical procedures, there is no institutional mechanism, no government pressure for health providers to act on the results of any evaluation done.[23] Thus, although John O'Brien-Bell may say that it is up to the government to decide how much high-tech care should be given, who is going to force hospitals and their heart bypass teams to be more judicious in selecting the patients they operate on?

Health Outcomes as Performance Standards

Let us turn now to the broader question of how well the health-care system is doing and consider some statistics. If you are a man aged 40 years, your life expectancy is no better than it was for your 40-year-old great-grandfather 100 years ago.[24] He had, and you have, a statistical chance of living another 34.3 years. This fact may seem hard to believe, because we keep hearing how more people are living longer thanks to the wonders of medical science. It is a fact often cited by medical authorities to justify the increasing cost of high-tech medicine. So is there a contradiction in this static expected lifespan of a 40-year-old male?

The contradiction is apparent rather than real, because we are used to hearing life expectancy values expressed for a one-minute-old infant. Life expectancy for babies at birth is indeed better today than it was 100 years ago, because infant mortality is lower, and childhood diseases kill very few children compared to the last century when children succumbed in droves to dysentery, diphtheria, measles and other infectious diseases. But once our nineteenth-century ancestors reached adulthood, threat of dying from infectious disease receded, and they lived the relatively healthy lives we experience today. And as I have said earlier, this was an era when there was no high-tech medicine and doctors believed in a hands-off approach.

Life expectancy values are simple mathematical exercises. Take a hypothetical case of two infants just born: one dies immediately and the other eventually lives to age 70. The life expectancy of the two at birth is the average – 35. If both infants live to age 70, their life expectancy at birth is 70, a dramatic doubling. Thus keeping more children alive until they reach adulthood has the statistical effect of raising life expectancy.

Life expectancy, in fact, is a crude index of health because individuals may survive many years in poor health, their quality of life slowly ebbing away. Two Canadian scientists feel that a better index is needed, one that gives some measure of life's quality rather than just its length. Russell Wilkins, an anthropologist at the Institute for Research on Public Policy in Montreal, and Owen Adams, a statistician at Statistics Canada, Ottawa, asked whether or not Canadians are healthier now than formerly. Is there less sickness than before? Using the same statistical methods used to calculate life expectancy, they constructed a *health expectancy index* that tells you how long you can expect to live before some disabling disease or condition impairs your functioning.[25]

Their index, in effect, takes overall life expectancy and breaks it into two parts: years of disability-free life and years of disabled life. Wilkins and Adams, in applying their index to Canadians over the 27-year period 1951–78, found that a Canadian male born in 1951 could look forward to living to age 60 before becoming disabled while a female born in that year would reach 65. When they looked at Canadians' health twenty-five years later in 1978, they found the health expectancy had barely budged, by only a 1.3 year extension of disability-free time. During the same period, the life expectancy from birth shot up some 4.5 years.

In other words, Canadians live longer from birth but live a larger part of their lives in a disabled state. There is no reason to believe that the health expectancy values are much different for populations of other industrialized countries. Wilkins and Adams, in fact, noted that there has been a 25 per cent increase in long-term disability among Americans.

The Iron Triangle

The critical analysis of life expectancy statistics by Wilkins and Adams lends support to Wildavsky's comment that medical care has a marginal effect on the overall health of the population. Yet governments remained locked into a policy of fostering access to high-tech medical care. Why should this be so in the face of evidence that it is not at all that successful and there are alternatives? There is an expression in Washington DC, 'the iron triangle' which refers to a three-cornered alliance that promotes a special interest at the expense of the common good. It consists of an industry, the bureaucrats who oversee the industry, and the politicians who make policy governing the industry. Such a triangle surely operates in the health sector. The medical–industrial complex is triangulated with the bureaucrats of the health agencies and the politicians who have a vested interest in making health appropriations.

The health-care iron triangle is a master at defending its special interests, suppressing any claim that its high technology is over applied and under effective. The name may be American, but such triangulated vested interests dominate the health-care systems of all industrialized countries.

This iron triangle, with its hermetically sealed interests, deflects any interest in acid rain, ocean decay, smog and alternative roads to health. There are indeed critics within and without the health-care system who would like to open government health policy to prevention, but it is unlikely that the system itself will recognize opportunities for improving the health of populations through social measures and arresting the decline in environmental quality.

5

Big Cancer

Chinese cooking can be hazardous to your lungs: that is, if you are a Chinese woman and stand every day over a fuming wok. Chinese women have the same rate of lung cancer as American women but, according to William Blot, chief of the biostatistics branch of the United States National Cancer Institute (NCI), only about one quarter of the Chinese cancer is due to cigarette smoking.[1] He believes that the smoke from the cooking oil is responsible for the high incidence of the disease. The cooking oil itself is not carcinogenic, but in the high heat of the wok it undergoes a chemical reaction forming volatile, cancer-causing substances. On the plus side, Blot said, eating fresh vegetables, particularly Chinese cabbage and other Chinese greens, lowers the risk of all forms of cancer.

There are factors, it seems, in one's ordinary environment that either cause or prevent cancer, and in fact, the risk of getting cancer is one of the fears people most often raise with respect to toxic substances in the environment. Cancer should, then, be a strong motivating force for cleaning up the environment, but it does not seem to have worked out that way. That statement may seem odd in view of the high profile cancer enjoys in the public eye, but the fact that fear of cancer has not brought about more noticeable results illustrates the difficulty of harnessing a public health issue to drive environmental protection.

There is certainly strong motivation for eliminating cancer. Armand Hammer, chairman of Occidental Petroleum Corporation and chairman of the President's Cancer Panel, believes cancer can be cured by the year 2000 if sufficient money is pumped into the scientific community. Hammer is convinced that the cure for cancer is just over the horizon and that the more money spent on the search the faster we will get to the cure. 'The price of delay is unacceptable,' Hammer says. 'Each year, this disease affects one out of three Americans and kills 500,000, almost as many as were killed in World War II, the Korean War and Vietnam combined. The longer we wait, the greater the toll will be.'[2]

NCI (just one of many cancer organizations in the industrialized countries), already spends $1.5 billion of taxpayers' money a year on cancer research and Hammer wants to increase that sum to $2.5 billion. Hammer's view that spending more money searching for a cure is the way to deal with cancer reflects the official view of governments and medical authorities. Emphasis on search for a cure eclipses official interest in cancer prevention: yet not completely, by any means, because some steps towards prevention are being taken.

In 1984 NCI announced a plan to cut cancer deaths in the United States in half by the year 2000 by persuading people to alter just two lifestyle factors: stop smoking and lower consumption of fatty foods. The preventive stance of NCI is not as vigorous as it looks on the surface. Critics of the plan say: why single out just two factors, what about the chemical contaminants in the environment that are thought to cause cancer? They fault cancer authorities for a timid approach to prevention. But NCI feels it is on firm ground in making these recommendations. There is good evidence that fatty foods contribute to breast cancer, and the only people who don't believe that smoking causes lung cancer are executives of tobacco companies. Moreover, the recommendations are for lifestyle change and are personal. It is an individual choice, and if you come down with lung cancer, the government can say it warned you. Toxic chemicals in the environment that contribute to cancer, on the other hand, lie beyond the individual's powers of avoidance and, therefore, require broader intervention into society's lifestyle as a whole.

Governments are reluctant to embark upon such broad intervention because they claim that they haven't evidence of links between exposure to specific toxic chemicals in the environment and cancer. Without firm evidence, they say, they cannot justify elimination of the toxic chemicals. But, paradoxically, while claiming the absence of specific links, governments through their cancer agencies, such as NCI, do not encourage the preventive type of research that would identify such links. Samuel Epstein, a toxicologist specializing in the toxicity of environmental pollutants, in his book *The Politics of Cancer* estimates that no more than 12 per cent of NCI's budget goes to research on ways to prevent cancer. The other 88 per cent is devoted to search for a cure.[3]

Another person who decries the imbalance is Jan Stjernsward, chief of cancer control at the World Health Organization. Speaking at a 1986 world conference of cancer specialists in Budapest, Hungary, he said he could not understand why nations continue to spend most or all of their cancer budgets on treatment of patients and on a search for a cure: 'Only minimal resources are being allocated for prevention and early detection.' Yet, in Stjernsward's view, one third of all human cancers are preventable.[4]

Stjernsward's audience of cancer specialists from around the world was living testimony to what he was saying. Practically the entire audience was committed to finding a cure for cancer. The training and motivation of these specialists left them unreceptive to what the WHO official had to say about prevention. Why should all these specialists avoid research on prevention and do research that bears on cure for cancer? Undoubtedly, the specialists find their search for a cure professionally rewarding, but that is only part of the reason. The lack of scientists and other specialists working on ways to prevent cancer is evidence of the reality of the golden rule: he who has the gold makes the rules. The heavy bias towards cure is government policy, and that policy provides funds to train cure-oriented cancer workers, not prevention-oriented workers. So it is no wonder that Stjernsward was speaking to an audience of closed minds.

Why are governments so committed to cure rather than prevention of cancer? Cancer is an excruciatingly emotional issue and governments are expected to do something about it. As already mentioned, intervening into social and industrial practices to prevent cancer, in a politician's view, is like walking into a minefield. An unexpected issue can blow up at any moment and destroy the politician. So why walk into a minefield if you don't have to? Cure is a technological fix that does not require social intervention and is thus politically satisfying. Leave it to the scientists and doctors – never mind whether or not a cure is found; the government is seen to be doing its best to eliminate the scourge of cancer. That comment may seem cynical, but one has to have some appreciation what drives politicians, and wisdom is only a minor part of the drive.

I raised the question at the beginning of the book: What stops countries from rising to the Brundtland Commission's challenge to design preventive environmental strategies? Lack of motivation was one reason. Policy-makers have to feel the heat of the dragon's breath before they react, and it is obvious that politicians do not even see a cancer dragon in the form of toxic chemicals in the environment. This is not to suggest that the only motivation for cleaning up toxic chemicals should be to cut down the incidence of cancer. There are many other reasons for eliminating the chemicals, but the cancer threat appears in the public mind as one of the principal ones. And if there is no obvious threat, motivation for clean-up is feeble.

There are obviously contradictions here, so let us sort out some of the key elements in the cancer–environment story, beginning with the question: Is cancer really an environmental disease?

Is Cancer an Environmental Disease?

Is there really a cancer dragon in the environment? What does science tell us? John Higginson, a cancer epidemiologist and director of the WHO Centre for Research on Cancer in Lyons, concluded in the 1950s that 80–90 per cent of all cancer is caused by factors in the environment, and moreover, these are factors under human control. Thus cancer, according to Higginson, is theoretically preventable, if we identify and are able to deal with all these factors.

Environmental factors that cause cancer were, in fact, known long before this. As early as 1775, Percival Pott, a London physician, found that chimney sweeps had a high incidence of cancer of the scrotum as a result of their exposure to coal tars in the chimneys. (The chimney sweeps seldom changed their trousers or bathed.) And in this century, atomic radiation and ultraviolet rays from the sun were among the environmental factors to be identified as causing cancer. Higginson was the first scientist, however, to make such a sweeping connection of cancer with environmental factors, and in the thirty years since his first announcement, he and other scientists have amply confirmed his original conclusion.

Higginson defined the environment as one's total life experience. He included your marital status, what you eat, where you live, where you work, the air you breathe, the water you drink. Moreover, Higginson believed no single factor causes cancer but rather a constellation of factors interacting with each other.

Higginson was asked, some twenty-five years after he first announced his conclusions about environmental factors, why cancer scientists had not picked up his lead and started a search for precise identification of these factors. He replied: 'The idea of lifestyle is woolly and ill-defined and not expressible in scientific terms with the technology available. Most scientists, myself included, don't like something woolly.'[5]

'Woolly' is Higginson's word to express scientists' distaste for working with social and behavioural factors that cannot be reduced to hard scientific facts. When you talk of total life experience, you talk of a tangled mixture of human behaviour, social trends, environmental trends, government actions and industrial development. It is a messy morass when it comes to making a scientific study. There is nothing there that can be poured neatly into a test tube. What Higginson, in effect, acknowledges is that scientists are unable to develop a laboratory model of real life. Scientists prefer working in an abstract world of facts, theories and things that can be measured, a narrow world shorn of human factors. This is one reason why scientists prefer to search for the cancer cure. It is a world in which scientists feel comfortable, a world in which cancer is reduced to laboratory models: inbred mice that have cancer, cultures of cancer cells and, most recently, cancer genes. Scientists are convinced that such laboratory models will some day give them the clues to cure human cancer in the real world.

Many environmental advocates, curiously, have also opted for a narrow model of the world, but for a different reason. Their goal is clean-up of environmental pollution and, anxious for scientific support for their advocacy, they tapped Higginson's conclusions that cancer is an environmental disease. But they think of the environment in terms of air and water pollution, completely missing the totality in which Higginson uses the word *environment*. This is one reason why environmentalists have not been too successful in proving a cancer–pollution link.

It would be too simplistic, however, to suggest that narrow models of cancer are the main reason for an overwhelming bias towards treatment and cure. The type of research that Higginson describes as woolly, involving a combination of social factors, human behaviour, government policy and industrial planning, as well as the hard facts that come out of scientific laboratories, can be done. It is not done to any extent because few scientists are trained to do it. The vast sums of money poured into a search for the cure also have the effect of training young scientists to do this specialized research. Young college students entering graduate programmes find plenty of places in research laboratories to learn how to work with cancer models of mice, cell cultures and cancer genes, but hardly any places at all to learn how to develop preventive approaches.

'Woolly' studies can ask questions that make vested interests uncomfortable. NCI's modest proposal that United States citizens reduce fat in their diet and give up smoking met intense opposition from cattle producers (beef is cited as an example of fatty food). Evidence that smoking leads to lung cancer began to surface in the early 1950s – the evidence was not woolly; it was very convincing – yet the tobacco companies for thirty years fought a successful campaign to avoid curbs on tobacco advertising and restrictions on smoking in public places. Politicians joined in this rearguard action. Iain Macleod, British Minister of Health in 1966, for instance, said the government could not stand the loss of tobacco revenue, at that time £1 billion a year (it more than doubled by the 1980s). In short, any plan to improve the population's chances of remaining well through lifestyle changes can be stonewalled by politically powerful groups that feel threatened by those changes.

The search for a cancer cure is not going to threaten any established groups. Moreover, the search for a cure has built up its own powerful establishment around the world. This establishment consists of cancer research institutes, professional societies, university departments doing cancer research, hospitals, government agencies, all having a stake in keeping up the search for a cure.

The Rise of the American Cancer Establishment

The cancer establishment has grown in size and influence since the Second World War. Its growth has been no accident: that growth has been carefully charted and propelled by key individuals who believe that a cancer cure can be found if only enough effort is put into the search.

Some say the rapid and channelled growth of the cancer establishment started with Mary Lasker's cook. Mary Lasker was the wife of Albert Lasker, an advertising entrepreneur, who made enormous sums of money urging people to smoke Lucky Strikes ('Reach for a Lucky instead of a sweet'). Lasker set up the Albert and Mary Lasker Foundation in 1942 to support medical research. His wife, energetic and strong-willed, took charge of the foundation and used it as a base from which to wield her influence.[6] Cancer was the one disease that captured her attention; and not just the disease itself, but also the way it was handled in society at that time.

Her cook fell ill with cancer in 1943 and was isolated by her doctor in a 'home for incurables'. Brimming with annoyance by the way her cook was abandoned by the medical profession, Lasker contacted Clarence Little, head of the American Society for Control of Cancer. This voluntary society had, for the past decade, waged a publicity campaign exhorting the American people to 'Fight Cancer with Knowledge'. Lasker was unimpressed by this campaign and appalled by the lack of organization and drive in the society and by its puny budget. Used to the high-powered world of business with its hard deals and decisive actions, she and her husband set out to displace the medical doctors that then controlled this society.

She and a small group of business associates won control of the board from the doctors and renamed the society the American Cancer Society (ACS). Within two years the born again society increased its take from the American public fifty-fold. Lasker and her colleagues set the ACS on a course from which it has never wavered; the search for improved treatment of cancer patients and for the ultimate cure.

Lasker realized that for a volunteer society, like the ACS, to succeed, it had to have public support for its goals. The society started a major campaign, as one critic complained, that inspired fear of death and incited public panic. Indeed, through articles in *Reader's Digest*, *Life* and other prominent magazines as well as through pamphlets available in every doctor's office, ACS intoned the message: 'One in five of us – every fifth person – will die of cancer.'

The ACS has never stopped fanning public fears about cancer, which is now the most feared of all major diseases. Public donations have kept rolling in and the ACS has become a major – perhaps the major – policy-maker in the cancer field in the United States.

One reason for this dominance is its relationship with the government cancer institute, NCI. This institute was created by the United States federal government in 1937 as a unit of the National Institutes of Health, Bethesda, Maryland. NCI's brief was to engage in research into the causes and treatment of cancer. For the first decade of its existence, it puttered along on a minuscule budget, not much larger than that of ACS: $0.5 million in 1945. Moreover, NCI's research attracted little interest in the scientific community. Cancer research lay at the bottom of the scientific pecking order, and top scientists by and large avoided the field. All that changed when Lasker and her colleagues turned their attention to Washington and its deep pockets.

They skilfully lobbied Senators and Congressmen, particularly Senators Claude Pepper of Florida and Lister Hill of Alabama and Congressman John Fogarty of Rhode Island, who controlled the health appropriations committees. They made certain the public was aware of Congressmen who voted in favour of those appropriations – what politician would want to be seen voting against money to be used to conquer a killer disease? Lasker and her Congressional allies (Mary and her little lambs, some critics called them) also had a strong ally in James Shannon, director of the National Institutes of Health from 1955 to 1968. Shannon used every dollar appropriated to his institutes, including NCI, to expand their programmes. By the end of the Eisenhower years in 1960, NCI's annual budget was running at $110 million.

NCI's constituency extends beyond its own extensive laboratories and scientific staff: over half its budget is given out in the form of grants and contracts to scientists in universities and research institutes across the country. (Cancer research is no longer considered a weak science and top scientists, including many winners of a Nobel Prize, now work in the field.) These scientists and their institutions have a vested interest in the welfare of NCI. In fact, the biological and health-related departments of most major United States universities would collapse if NCI money were suddenly withdrawn. This fact is constantly pressed home to politicians from every state. So what started as a small but effective lobbying effort by Mary Lasker and her colleagues is now reinforced by a large, nationwide lobby of cancer institutes, universities and their alumni.

The alliance between the American Cancer Society and the National Cancer Institute works to the advantage of both. NCI remains the professional organization devoted to spending public funds on cancer research and treatment. ACS remains a highly visible voluntary organization that sets cancer policy and ensures the continuing appropriation for NCI. It is a remarkable arrangement and probably no other country in the world could mobilize such a vast effort devoted to a single health goal, treatment and cure of cancer.

Cancer Research: The Search for the Cure

The sheer weight of the cancer research establishment of the United States dominates the style of cancer treatment and research in other countries. Lasker and her allies set her cancer policy in motion in the 1940s when Europe was recovering from the war. By the time, ten or fifteen years later, when European countries were ready to devote resources and energy to cancer, the American lead was overwhelming. Consequently, cancer policies in European countries, in fact throughout the whole world, as Stjernsward of WHO laments, are firmly set in the direction of the ultimate cure.

This large army of cancer researchers is co-ordinated (controlled might be a better word) through central granting agencies in each country. You can see that control working in the United States through the operations of ACS and NCI. These agencies hand out money in the form of contracts and grants to researchers in universities and research institutes. The contracts and grants are given for research in certain areas. That is, the researcher receives the money only if he is willing to work in a specified narrow area of science and, of course, has the necessary scientific capability to do the research. If the researchers stray from the designated area of research the grants or contracts are cut off.

The channelling of money into precisely defined areas of research has the effect of moving those areas along more rapidly, but it also has the effect of discouraging adventures off the beaten path.

When the cancer establishment was small, its impact on university research was also relatively small, but now whole departments, particularly in the biological and medical sciences, depend on the largesse of ACS and NCI. E. J. Sylvester, in his book *Target Cancer*, quotes a Boston cancer specialist saying that if a simple and inexpensive replacement for chemotherapy were discovered, all United States medical schools would teeter on the edge of bankruptcy.[7] Chemotherapy is one of the orthodox areas for cancer research, and research and treatment with chemicals bring in carloads of money. University faculties thus have a strong incentive to keep up research in chemotherapy. There is an absence of incentive to explore other paths.

The narrowness of cancer research worries some critics. An editor of the journal *Cancer Control* complained that the grant money was leading research scientists into smaller and smaller corners of the biomedical research universe. Lewis Thomas wrote in his 1983 book *The Youngest Science* that the huge sums of government money given to universities was putting them 'into a subservient relationship to Washington'.[8] In another article, on the same issue, Thomas observed that the whole operation of cancer research has become too bureaucratic, too goal-directed. Bureaucratic plans 'fail to allow for the surprise which surely must lie ahead'.[9]

Surprises are a normal occurrence in unfettered science. Imagine a group of medical doctors in 1895 being asked to come up with a new diagnostic tool. It is unlikely that any of these medically trained doctors would have though of the X-ray, discovered by Wilhelm Roentgen, a physicist. Yet today narrowly trained scientists and medical doctors are being asked to 'conquer cancer'. Whether or not they will be successful is not the point I wish to make. The issue from the environmental perspective is that the bureaucratic direction of cancer research, seemingly cast in concrete in the mid-1940s, principally by Lasker and her colleagues, suppresses study of a broader, preventive approach to cancer.

John Cairns, an Australian cancer scientist, who sees cancer in its relationship to the kind of society we live in, states bluntly that failure to implement preventive measures is undermining US efforts to control cancer. 'None of the important causes of death has been primarily controlled by treatment,' Cairns says. 'The death rates from malaria, cholera, typhus, tuberculosis, scurvy, pellagra and other scourges of the past have dwindled in the US mainly because humankind has learned how to prevent these diseases, not simply because they can be treated.' Cairns adds: 'To put most of the effort into treatment is to deny all precedent'.[10]

Ironically, Higginson's original work on the environmental causes of cancer was done and the results widely circulated at the time Mary Lasker and ACS were setting out cancer policy. Serious health writers of the 1950s, in fact, picked up Higginson's results and wondered why ACS and NCI did not pay more attention to cancer as a *disease of civilization*. The Lasker group simply ignored the import of Higginson's studies, saying that research under their policy was on the verge of bringing forth a cure for cancer. Forty years later, cancer researchers are still on the verge.

Carcinogenesis

When Percival Pott, the London physician, observed the high rate of scrotal cancer in chimney sweeps, he said that there was something in coal tar that causes cancer. The idea that the human environment contains cancer-causing chemicals, called 'carcinogens', however, evolved slowly. One of the earlier proponents of this idea was Wilhelm Hueper, a German-born medical scientist. Hueper went to the United States in the 1920s to work for the Dupont Chemical Company. Aware that bladder cancer was frequent among workers in dye factories in Germany, Hueper studied workers in Dupont's dye plants. He found out that they too had a high incidence of bladder cancer caused by beta-naphthylamine, a chemical used to make dyes. Hueper told his superiors about these findings in 1938, but Dupont refused Hueper permission to publish the findings, saying that it was not the Corporation's responsibility to warn workers of such dangers. To boot, they fired Hueper.

Undiscouraged, Hueper continued to study carcinogens, and in 1948, NCI hired him to head its newly created Environmental Cancer Unit. At that time, very few chemicals used in industry had been tested to see whether or not they could cause cancer. Hueper tested 1,329 chemicals in laboratory animals within his first three years and found thirty-two to be carcinogenic.[11]

Hueper was not simply a laboratory scientist. He cared deeply about the social implications of what he was finding. Much to the chagrin of NCI, he went public, advocating the elimination of carcinogenic chemicals from the workplace and advancing what was then a heretical idea – that communities should be protected from discharge of toxic chemical waste. NCI tried to muzzle Hueper. They ordered him to cease all field work, that is, study of human cancers such as he had been conducting at Dupont. Finally, they exercised the golden rule and cut his budget. Experiments with animals are costly, and at a time when NCI's total budget was reaching the $100 million mark, the budget for Hueper's carcinogenic work totalled about $0.5 million, enough to conduct only a few animal experiments.

However, it was not just NCI that was trying to gag Hueper; the social climate of the 1940s and 1950s was hostile to this type of scientific research. James Patterson, a Harvard University historian, wrote in his book about the growth of the cancer establishment in the United States, *The Dread Disease*, that the government had no wish to alarm people about vague threats of environmental carcinogens.[12] The idea that there were man-made things in the environment that could be harmful was untenable.

Cornelius Rhodes, head of the prestigious Memorial Cancer Research Institute, New York, authoritatively pronounced that the atomic radiation from open-air atomic tests being conducted by the United States in the Pacific in the 1950s was harmless. Patterson comments that cancer scientists were not open to the idea that environmental factors played a significant role in causing the disease. He quotes a 1971 statement by Charles Cameron, scientific director of ACS, that the root cause of cancer is 'individual susceptibility' to the disease. Such thinking led to the belief that most preventive measures suggested were useless and could be socially disruptive.

Patterson also points out that the US political climate in the 1950s and 1960s was against environmental action: 'Tired of social reform they [Americans] showed little interest in erecting elaborate federal regulation of alleged polluters and in pointing accusatory fingers at industrial statesmen'.[13]

Cancer and the Environmental Movement

The environmental movement was not active during the early period when Mary Lasker and her allies set the cancer establishement on its course towards the cure. By the time the environmental movement emerged in the late 1960s and 1970s, its promotion of cancer prevention through environmental clean-up had to buck a large, entrenched cancer establishment dead set against wasting time trying to prevent cancer.

If environmentalists had been more forthright with the general public in terms of what the environmental hazards were, and downplayed the cancer angle, they would not have collided with the cancer establishment. As it is, they tried to siphon off some of the public fear of cancer for their own ends. Toxic chemicals in the environment can cause a lot of health problems, including increased birth defects, lowered intelligence, neurological deficit, and a drop in immune defences leading to increased susceptibility to a variety of ills in addition to cancer. By playing up the cancer threat alone, environmentalists wound up having to argue with the cancer establishment over whether or not chemical pollutants at the levels found in drinking water, air and food cause cancer. It is an argument the environmentalists lost, because by zeroing in on cancer, authorities could argue that the levels of toxic chemicals found in the environment are trivial and do not present a cancer risk. By keeping the argument on such a narrow path, environmentalists may well have set back progress in the control of chemical pollution.

The fear of cancer is certainly a legitimate fear, but it has not been placed in balance with other health threats. Rachel Carson was perhaps the first writer to exploit the fear of cancer. She was greatly influenced by Hueper's work and his conviction that carcinogenic substances in the environment are a serious threat. She devoted a chapter in her book *Silent Spring* to the carcinogenic effects of pesticides, writing of a 'sea of carcinogens', a sea that would cause cancer in 45 million Americans living today.[14] She noted that some carcinogens are natural, such as the ultraviolet rays of sunlight, but claimed that most carcinogens were man-made.

Samuel Epstein wrote in *The Politics of Cancer* that industrial pollution accounted for 30–40 per cent of cancers.[15] And Larry Agran, a lawyer specializing in environmental issues, published another widely circulated book in which he predicted a 'cancer pox' and the 'unmistakable emergence of a national cancer epidemic' which would kill three out of four Americans.[16] Not all those in the environmental movement took such extreme positions, but there was general agreement that cancer is an environmentally caused disease and that chemical pollution is a principal cause. Higginson's work was often quoted to back up these claims, a fact that annoyed Higginson. In an interview with Thomas Maugh of *Science* magazine in 1979, Higginson said, 'I'm all for cleaning up the air, and all for cleaning up trout streams, and all for preventing Love Canals, but I don't think we should use the wrong argument for doing it. To make cancer the whipping boy for every environmental evil may prevent effective action when it does matter, as with cigarettes.'[17] Higginson went on to say, 'people would love to be able to prove that cancer is due to pollution in the general environment', because then all we would have to do is to regulate chemicals out of the environment and 'we have no more cancer'. Higginson found this logic simplistic. He said that chemical pollution may indeed be part of the cancer problem, but it was only part and that there are other reasons for cleaning up pollution.[18]

So when it comes to raising the panic level, the environmentalists were as guilty as ACS of fanning public fear of cancer and raising public expectations. Whereas ACS held out a vision of a laboratory cure just around the corner, environmentalists held out a vision of a chemical-free environment as the ultimate solution. Their solution was better than a cure, because people would not get cancer.

Where is the truth in these claims? I will come to the soon-to-arrive cancer cure in a moment. What of the 'sea of carcinogens?' There is, of course, an element of truth in this idea. Hueper's pioneering work did indeed point out the carcinogenic nature of a lot of chemical pollutants to which we are exposed. Ironically, if Hueper and other scientists studying chemical carcinogens had been given more support in the 1940s and 1950s, we would have had a more rounded understanding of this cause of cancer by the time the environmental movement began to grab public attention in the 1970s. As it was, when Carson, Epstein and others were talking about a sea of carcinogens, knowledge of chemical carcinogenesis was fragmentary, with just enough known to make the concept of a cancer-causing sea of environmental contaminants plausible.

Our knowledge of chemical carcinogenesis is not much better now. The subject continues to enjoy as much popularity at NCI as it did in Hueper's time. Of some 100,000 chemicals used in commerce – the majority of which wind up in the environment in some way – only about 5 per cent have ever been tested thoroughly to find out if they cause cancer. That leaves a lot of room, as Lewis Thomas said, for surprises about environmental exposure to chemicals and cancer.

In any event, we know enough to suggest, as Higginson says, that while exposure to chemical contaminants should be minimized, we should not try to pin the cancer problem exclusively on chemical pollution. Higginson notes that the amount of cancer on a per capita basis in Birmingham, England, an industrial area of high pollution, is lower than that of Geneva, Switzerland, a relatively industry-free city. Leaders in the environmental movement have damaged their cause by stressing a cancer–pollution link because their arguments are easily rebutted by comparisons such as that between Birmingham and Geneva. Moreover, in an attempt to buttress their argument with hard, scientific data, environmentalists often claim that a single chemical is a dangerous cancer hazard.

Too much emphasis is placed on *the* cause of cancer. Too much time is wasted arguing over whether a single substance causes or does not cause cancer, rather than looking at multiple causes. Higginson talks of a plurality of factors. Cancer in most instances results from a constellation of factors: air pollutants, what you eat and drink, and lifestyle factors, such as whether you are single or married. It is a muddled, woolly situation, and so far, environmentalists, cancer scientists and public health policy-makers all shy away from addressing the muddle and woolliness that is real life.

Unbalanced Cancer Research

I would like to come back to Armand Hammer and his billion-dollar crusade against cancer. Hammer was ninety years old when, in 1988, he announced his lifetime goal: cure cancer by his hundredth birthday. Hammer, no lightweight in business and government policy-making circles, said in interview that the cancer crusade had become the central part of his life. 'It takes priority over everything.'[19]

One of the ironic aspects of Hammer's quest for a cancer cure is that as majority owner of Occidental Petroleum Company he is alo owner of its subsidiary, Occidental Chemical Company, Niagara Falls, NY: the chemical company, formerly Hooker Chemicals, best known as the creator of the Love Canal waste dump. Occidental Petroleum's contributions to Hammer's initiative thus derive in part from the profits of its chemical subsidiary. The company has a poor record in general concerning the dumping of toxic chemicals into the environment and has been cited by Greenpeace as one of the 'filthy five' industries of the United States.

In any event, gold is gold, and cancer researchers are ecstatic at the prospect of bigger grants, although some have reservations about how the money will be allocated. Hammer believes that the cure for cancer will be found in the narrow field of immunology, the idea that people can be immunized against cancer. Critics worry that much of this new money will wind up drawing cancer researchers into Hammer's pet research field.

There is a tendency for cancer scientists and policy-makers, like Hammer, to jump on bandwagons when a particular field of science is going well – as immunology is at the moment. But bandwagons break down. Albert Tannenbaum, the 1957 president of the professional organization, American Association for Cancer Research, berated his fellow researchers for climbing on one bandwagon after another: transplantation therapy, immunology, carcinogenesis, enzyme activity, chemotherapy, new diagnostic tests. Tannenbaum, like Lewis Thomas, recognized that we do not know enough about cancer to predict how – if ever – it can be cured. Cancer research, in his view, should be spread over many fields. Now, thirty years later, the same worry has surfaced in face of Hammer's impending gift. David Korn, dean of Stanford University medical school and chairman of an advisory group for NCI, was particularly unsettled by the ten-year goal, saying that it would raise the expectations of the public: 'I don't believe and I don't think anybody believes that having another several hundred million dollars over the next few years is going to assure some magical result in cancer control disease prevention or anything else.'[20]

Cancer research has indeed, since Mary Lasker set the course for cure, made great advances, as publicists for cancer societies are forever pointing out. But this new knowledge has not made much of a dent in the cancer statistics. The number of new cases each year and the death rate from cancer in the USA have remained about the same for the last thirty years. In fact, the number of new cases may be going up, according to a report from NCI released in 1988. Lung cancer cases (as expected) continue to mount as the teenagers who started smoking around the time of the Second World War reach their fifties and sixties. But what surprised officials was that the number of cases of other major forms of cancer, such as breast cancer, is rising at about 1 per cent a year.[21]

Hammer is convinced that the only reason that we do not yet have a cancer cure is lack of money. But cancer is elusive, like exploring a large mansion in the dark. We do not know how large the cancer mansion is. In spite of the billions spent on research, for all we know we may still have explored only the foyer. Lewis Thomas, more than anyone, has the ability to throw cold water on those who trumpet that the big cancer breakthrough is about to happen. Give us a billion dollars a year and we will cure cancer within ten years, NCI officials said in 1974 when announcing their plan of funnelling cancer research into areas they designated as the breakthrough fields. Thomas quietly pointed out: 'It seems to us a defect of the [NCI] cancer plan is that the enormity of our ignorance about cancer receives less emphasis than it merits.'[22]

In spite of such reservations, the cancer establishment, now mature, fantastically wealthy and with a rhinoceros hide when it comes to responding to criticism, remains wedded to the idea of research into cure, and that is where the money goes and where public prestige lies. This establishment has successfully focused public and government attention on its agenda. One casualty of that focus is failure to develop a systematic effort to prevent cancer, an effort that surely would boost the drive to clean up the environment. In short, the motivation to deal with the cancer problem is strong, but very little of that motivation is pointed towards prevention.

Part II

Environment and the Preventive Approach

6

Risk Assessment: Is it Appropriate for Environmental Action?

This is a transitional chapter in which the focus shifts from health-care attitudes and policies to environmental issues. In this chapter we begin to see how the health-care system – the medical–industrial complex, the individual doctors, the politicians, the health bureaucrats, the consumers of health-care – influences the way we go about identifying environmental ills and how we try to correct them.

From much of what has been recounted in previous chapters, the health-care system would be expected to have little influence one way or the other, given the indifference among health-care professionals, preoccupied as it were with their task of curing the nation's health problems. But on the contrary, the influence is marked, and what this second part of the book does is show how that influence retards development of a strong environmental policy – the kind of policy Brundtland looks for.

The reason for this influence is that environmental actions are driven by threats to human health and well-being. Very few government actions towards protecting the environment are launched that are not perceived as addressing a threat to people's health. All pesticide regulations, for example, are based on the threat of pesticide residues to humans, not to other species. And this is one of the reasons why environmental decisions fall so short of meeting the actual problems confronting us.

Although human health drives environmental action, the driving force lacks vigour and conviction. It is like putting a lawn mower engine in a racing car: it's an engine of sorts, but hardly adequate. Brundtland touches on this point in her dismissal of government environmental bureaucracies as ill-equipped to deal with the problems of world decay. One reason they are ill-equipped is that environmental bureaucrats try to extend medical approaches to the way they deal with problems of the environment. In this transitional chapter we look at how a tool of medical diagnosis – risk assessment – has become the principal way of assessing the nature and extent of environmental ills.

Assessment of Risk of Heart Attack

Medical students have hammered into them the belief that you cannot deal with a problem if you do not know what it is, and diagnosis, indeed, is the prime function of the clinician. All very well, but, as pointed out earlier, medical doctors operate according to the one-cause/one-effect thinking of the biomedical model, and it is this kind of diagnostic thinking intended for use in doctors' surgeries that is extended to environmental issues. Risk assessment is very much a one-cause/one-effect exercise.

What is risk assessment and how do doctors use it? Suppose you regularly eat large T-bone steaks, french fries with ketchup and loads of ice cream. It is doubtful that your diet would convince your doctor that a long, disease-free life stretches ahead of you. The doctor will be even less convinced if she takes a blood sample and finds that your cholesterol level is elevated. If she is like many doctors, she considers that this style of eating increases the risk of suffering a heart attack, and the elevated cholesterol is proof of the increased risk.

It is worth pursuing the cholesterol–heart connection further, to see how risk assessment is used to assess one's health. The human arterial system, expecially in the heart arteries, is prone to buildup of plaques, a mixture of cholesterol and fat. As mentioned earlier, one way of treating the buildup is to have a heart bypass operation, but operation or not, the stage is set for disaster. Clots form in the arteries from time to time, and for a normally unblocked artery, a clot passes on through harmlessly; but for an artery partially blocked with plaques, the clot may stick in the narrowed opening. Blood flow stops suddenly, precipitating the heart attack. The heart muscle is supplied by several arteries and usually the blockage occurs in only one of them. It is as if an eight-cylinder engine is reduced to five or four cylinders: the heart may stop working or it may be able to continue, and with rest and treatment the damaged tissue heals and the individual recovers.

Not all people develop atherosclerosis, and for those who do, the rate at which the plaques grow varies enormously. Some individuals may suffer a heart attack at age thirty-five or forty, while others have them in their sixties and seventies. So this is where risk assessment comes in: the likelihood of having a heart attack depends on the likelihood of the plaques growing to the extent where they block 50 per cent or more of the cross-sectional area of a coronary artery. The indicator chosen by medical science to predict the likelihood of plaque formation and a heart attack is the level of cholesterol in one's blood. Why cholesterol?

The theory of atherosclerosis, in its simplest form, is that large scavenger cells lining the coronary arteries, called macrophages, engulf excess cholesterol from the blood. The engorged macrophages release chemical factors that cause cells in the arterial walls to divide. The net result: a jumbled mound of cells, cholesterol and other fats start to build up – a plaque. The whole process seems to be triggered and sustained by an elevated blood cholesterol level. Thus, theory states, the higher the level of cholesterol in the blood, the more plaque formation is stimulated. Consequently the risk of a heart attack is greater.

There is another reason for choosing blood cholesterol level as an indicator: practicality. Total blood cholesterol is easily measured. A doctor can buy and install a machine in her surgery that measures total cholesterol in a few minutes – giving her a scale on which to judge the fate of her patients. The National Cholesterol Education Program, run by the National Heart, Lung and Blood Institute, Bethesda, Maryland, set 200 mg/dl as the threshold limit for safety.[1] Individuals with levels between 200 and 239 are considered borderline high risk, and anyone with a count of 240 or more is at high risk. In other words, the risk is quantified in numbers easily understood by doctors and their patients. More than one third of American men have blood cholesterol levels of 240 or higher, which is what the Cholesterol Education Program wishes to correct.[2]

Blood cholesterol levels can be lowered by cutting down on fatty foods, meat, eggs and dairy products and by engaging in regular exercise. For those who find lifestyle change difficult, new drugs are entering the market. They are able to lower the level of blood cholesterol, and most importantly, seem to lower the risk of a heart attack. One such drug, gemfibrozil (Lopid), sold by Parke Davis & Company, was studied in 4,081 middle-aged men in Finland. For five years, half the men took the drug while the other half took a placebo. It was what is called a double blind trial; neither the men nor their doctors knew who took the drug and who took the placebo. The code which listed drug-takers and placebo takers was broken only after the five-year period was up, revealing that the drug-takers suffered 34 per cent fewer heart attacks.[3] Supported by such results, highly publicized, the market for such drugs is bullish. Sales of cholesterol-lowering drugs in the United States in 1988 were $304 million and are expected to exceed $1 billion by 1992.[4]

Like all aspects of scientific medicine, assessment of the risk of heart attacks is based on the biomedical model. The essence of the model is diagnosis of a health problem in a one-to-one relationship: the assessment of the risk of suffering a heart attack is, in fact, a diagnosis, relating the outcome to something that can be analysed, namely cholesterol. A critical point in making such a diagnosis is that there must be hard scientific evidence of the relationship. Evidence linking blood cholesterol level and risk of heart attacks has been slow in coming. For the past thirty-five years the link has been suspected, but it has taken a very large corps of scientific investigators in all industrialized countries, spending more than a billion dollars a year, to confirm it. Yet, in spite of all this time and effort expended, medical opinion is by no means unanimous that total blood cholesterol is that significant an indicator of the risk of having a heart attack. One sceptic, Robert Olson, professor of medicine at the State University of New York, Stony Brook, claims that 200 mg/dl is not a magic threshold. He says, 'there is no convincing evidence that 199mg/dl is less risky than 210mg/dl.' He also notes that in the drug intervention trials (like the Finnish study) a slight reduction in mortality due to heart disease shows up, but that overall mortality does not change.[5] In other words, individuals die of other causes, adverse effects of the drug being a contributing factor. Olson is sceptical of the value of giving blanket advice about diet and other lifestyle factors to a large segment of the population with the promise that heart disease will thereby be avoided.

The onset of heart disease is undoubtedly more complex than suggested by the elevated cholesterol theory. Monkeys and rats fed a high-cholesterol diet contract atherosclerosis just like humans, but a series of experiments carried out in the 1960s showed that when the animals received extra vitamin B6, or lethicin, atherosclerosis did not occur.[6] These experiments seem to have been forgotten in the current rage over cholesterol.

Whether or not blood cholesterol accurately reveals the state of one's personal biology, however, is beside the point: the health-care system has made it an important indicator for risk assessment, a tool for advocating behavioural changes in people's lives. But is such risk assessment the kind of tool government bureaucrats should be using to assess the state of ecological systems?

How do you Cook a Poisoned Goose?

Let us look at how risk assessment was applied to one ecological system: the fields and streams of Montana with their ducks and geese and their hunters. The specific problem: What is the risk of eating a goose contaminated with the pesticide, Endrin? Endrin is a highly toxic and persistent pesticide widely used by Montana farmers. The pesticide is sprayed from aircraft and covers not only crop areas but large areas of countryside inhabited by flocks of ducks and geese. Over the spring and summer these waterfowl eat the pesticide-contaminated vegetation and by the time the autumn hunting season rolls around they have built up a high concentration of Endrin in their flesh. The pesticide is just as persistent in the birds as in the vegetation.

Now the dilemma. The Montana government was reluctant to ban hunting of the toxic birds because of the popularity of the sport. They could not suggest that the hunters simply throw the killed birds away, because State law makes it a crime not to eat any bird shot. They could have banned Endrin, but a coalition of farmers and Endrin's manufacturers lobbied successfully against the ban, saying Montana farmers could not compete without using the pesticide.

The bureaucrats of the State Department of Fish, Wildlife and Parks, according to *Sierra* magazine,[7] hit upon a solution – instruct hunters how to cook a toxic goose: (1) Trim all fat from goose and discard skin and internal organs in an approved toxic waste disposal site. (2) Fully cook the skinned bird on a rack and also discard the drippings in the approved toxic waste disposal site. (3) Do not stuff the bird. (4) Pregnant family members and women contemplating pregnancy should not eat the fowl. (No mention of men contemplating fathering.) (5) Do not eat more than one duck or one pound of goose per week, a maximum of six ducks or six pounds of goose per hunting season.

This is the kind of risk assessment practised by bureaucrats towards environment: messy and pragmatic. It is messy because of the uncertainty as to the amount of Endrin in the ducks, the amount of exposure of duck eaters and the health effects on the eaters. It is pragmatic because no vested interest is stepped on – not the pesticide maker, nor farmers, nor gun-makers, nor hunters – and the recommendations, in spite of the uncertainty of exposure and health effects, are given in precise, no-nonsense terms – six ducks or six pounds of goose per season, cooked according to the State recipe.

In actual fact, the uncertainty makes the whole exercise a guessing game. What happens if you eat more than six ducks? No one knows or, for that matter, will ever know. The scientific research is not there. Montana authorities have no extensive knowledge base from which to back their prediction of the fate of people who eat more than six ducks.

But the authorities were not completely without information. We know that Endrin is a toxic chemical, so why is there so much uncertainty about the effects on humans exposed to it? The answer to this question spotlights the difficulty of making risk assessments about chemicals in the environment. And bear in mind that we are talking here of assessing the risk of a single chemical. The assumption has to be made that the individual is exposed to no other chemical, which may be quite unrealistic in view of total exposure to environmental contaminants in food, water and air.

Nevertheless, bureaucrats make risk assessments on single chemicals, so let us assess the knowledge base which they use to determine how dangerous a pesticide like Endrin is. To start you have to know two things: the toxicity of the substance (that is, how much of the substance does it take to poison an animal or human and what form does the poisoning take – liver damage, heart failure, brain damage and so on); and degree of exposure. Strychnine is extremely toxic, but as long as it is contained in a bottle it poses no threat. But if it is in your porridge...! Toxicologists use the term hazard to denote a combination of the toxicity of a substance and the degree of exposure to it. A very toxic substance and a small degree of exposure can be just as hazardous as a slightly toxic substance and a large degree of exposure.

This sounds straightforward enough, but the uncertainty in risk assessment, which is supposed to assign a number to the hazard (e.g., one's risk of cancer is 1 in 10,000) comes about because of an inability to quantify precisely either exposure or toxicity. As we saw in the case of Montana ducks, you can make only a broad-brush guess about exposure; and although science has made startling strides in many fields, toxicology is not one of them.

Toxicology: A Laboratory Science, not a Field Science

The science of toxicology presents environmental decision-makers with two deficiencies: first, environmental problems are out in the field, where problems like that of ducks and Endrin exist, whereas toxicology remains a practice of the laboratory; and the methods toxicology uses date from scientific antiquity, the remarkable developments in biotechnology over the past three decades having passed it by. It is these deficiencies that make diagnosis of environmental ills with risk assessment at best superficial.

Here is what one noted biologist thought about toxicology. Donald Kennedy, President of Stanford University and formerly Head of the Food and Drug Administration (FDA), Washington DC, said that of all the biological disciplines, 'only nutrition approaches toxicology in terms of being basically in bad shape.'[8] While at the FDA Kennedy was frustrated by the antiquated methods toxicologists use to determine the toxicity of food additives and drugs: methods that never give precise information, leaving the door open for interpretation according to one's particular vested interest. This is one reason why so many drugs are initially approved by the FDA as being safe, only to be found later to injure or kill patients.

Since environmental bureaucrats base so many policy decisions on the science of toxicology, it is worth taking a moment to look further into what information the science can give and to see how relevant it is to environmental issues. We need to keep in mind that risk assessment in the environment requires knowing both exposure and toxicity: the science of toxicology, even if it gave superlative, unequivocal answers, would still have nothing to say about exposure in the field.

One of the reasons for the shakiness of toxicity data is that toxicologists rely heavily on experiments with animals – rats, mice and sometimes larger animals such as cats, dogs and monkeys. Each animal is an individual and responds differently to a chemical being tested. To get around that problem scientists give groups of test animals given doses of the chemical. At a specific dose, for example, five out of ten animals may die, the other five remain perfectly healthy. At a lower dose maybe only one animal dies. This is what scientists call a dose/response curve. If you give enough of the chemical the response is death. If you give enough arsenic to a rich uncle, the uncle dies. You do not have to be a scientist to observe the effect of arsenic at the high end of the dose/response curve. But at the low end of the curve, toxic effects are much more difficult to pinpoint.

Yet it is the low end of the dose/response curve that interests environmental regulators. Is there a low enough level below which arsenic ceases to be toxic? That is the question, because if you are a bureaucrat responsible for setting the safe level of arsenic in drinking water, you need to know the threshold and set a water standard below that point. Toxicology fails to provide a precise threshold.

A lot of confusion and argument swirls around thresholds. There are, in fact, dozens of thresholds for any one chemical in an experimental animal. Each possible toxic effect, from liver damage to reproductive damage, has a threshold. The threshold for damage to the immune system might be at a level 1,000 or 10,000 times lower than that for liver damage. So, from the point of view of risk assessment, what threshold are we talking about? To add to the confusion, there are experts who argue that for some effects like cancer, there is no threshold. And to top it all, toxicologists are unable to test for every conceivable effect that might occur. Thus, even when a safety threshold is set, based on laboratory data, a chemical may still have harmful effects below that threshold.

It is very difficult to obtain full information. The US National Academy of Sciences carried out a survey of all pesticides now approved for use; these chemicals presumably had been thoroughly studied, but the Academy found that for not one of them (and most are in wide use) was the information about toxicity complete.[9]

I do not wish to leave the impression that the science of toxicology is unhelpful. It can provide a lot of basic information about the toxicity of a chemical and as long as you accept the limitations of the laboratory data and the gaps in those data, the information can be useful. Toxicology, in fact, works reasonably well at the higher ends of the dose/response curve, for example at the level of a chemical in a factory to which workers might be exposed, or in police cases, such as poisoned uncles. But its very success in these situations gives the science more credibility than it deserves when it comes to assessing the hazard of long-term, low-level exposure, which is the case of environmental contamination.

Toxicologists Test Single Chemicals

Throughout this exposition of toxicology it should be obvious that there is one fatal flaw in the science from the environmental perspective: toxicologists test only one chemical at a time. All the information that we have (such as it is) is obtained on single chemicals. In the field, the environment where we all live, we are exposed to a multitude of toxic chemicals, pesticide residues in our food, contaminants in our drinking water, chemicals in every breath of air; all this adds up to a total toxic exposure. Long-term exposure, we know, can lead to a variety of effects: cancer, depressed immune system, malaise that defies medical diagnosis or birth defects passed on to succeeding generations. The science of toxicology is unable to predict what, if anything, this environmental exposure will cause in each of us.

We have a paradox: the real world is multiple chemicals, long-term exposure at low dose; the laboratory world is single chemicals in high doses. It is a paradox that reveals the leverage of medical science and the health-care system. The environmental community, when challenged by the problem of assessing environmental exposure of toxic chemicals, has chosen not to accept the challenge; instead, it has adopted the medical world's way of looking at nature and opted for risk assessment of environmental contaminants one at a time. In other words, there has been no attempt to develop a new science capable of examining the health effects of multiple toxic chemicals under the conditions found in the environment.

The one-cause/one-effect nature of risk assessment leads to anomalous conclusions, illustrated by this assessment of the risk of eating a mushroom – not the poisonous kind you might mistakenly pick in the woods, but the safe kind you buy in the supermarket. Bruce Ames, a biochemist at the University of California at Berkeley, has developed a scheme for ranking the cancer risk from things to which humans are commonly exposed to. You cannot, of course, develop such an assessment by experimenting with humans, but Ames feels that experiments conducted in laboratory rats and mice can be used to rank the power of chemicals to cause cancer in humans. Chemicals vary greatly in their power to cause cancer in laboratory animals. Ames finds that some chemicals are 10 million times more potent than others. Moreover, he notes that in our normal life we are exposed to many natural substances that cause cancer in rodents, as well as to man-made chemicals. He cites common plants used for food which contain toxic substances to protect them against fungi, viruses and insects. Many such components also happen to cause cancer, and Ames includes these natural substances in his scale of cancer risk.[10]

Ames takes tap water as his base and estimates that if you eat one peanut butter sandwich a day, your risk of cancer is thirty times that incurred by drinking one litre of tap water per day. Eating one raw mushroom a day is 100 times as risky, and drinking one can of beer a day is 2,800 times as risky, while a quarter bottle of wine a day ups the risk 4,700 times over tap water. And for those taking the cholesterol-lowering drug, Clofibrate, the risk skyrockets to 17,000 times.

The numbers can be beguiling, for they teeter on a pile of assumptions. First of all, as Ames himself noted, the cancer-causing potency of these substances is determined in rats and mice and one has to assume that humans have the same degree of susceptibility. But further, Ames does not actually feed rats the peanut butter sandwiches, mushrooms or beer. He bases his estimates on known cancer-causing agents in these foods. Mushrooms contain a chemical called hydrazine, and it is the pure hydrazine that is tested in rats. But how do we know that when we eat a mushroom the hydrazine it contains will not act differently? Perhaps there are substances in the mushroom that cancel the effect of hydrazine, or for that matter, increase its cancer-causing potency. We do not know. Besides, what nutrition do you get from a bottle of hydrazine?[11]

Scientists love numbers, and quantitative differences are indeed helpful when the underlying data are sound. But the truth is that science lacks the means to assess the risk of disease from one's entire nutritional environment. So instead we have experiments with hydrazine, and to assign a number 30 to one mushroom per day on this basis makes as much sense as conducting the experiment on a roulette wheel.

Taking risk assessment out of the doctor's surgery and applying it to the environment leads to other anomalies. Bureaucrats who regulate pesticides and other environmental contaminants use risk assessment as a tool for cost/benefit analyses. They will say, yes, that chemical is risky, but what is the economic cost of banning it? Since the only biological species considered in doing a cost/benefit analysis is the human, it is necessary to attach a value to one human life. According to *Time* magazine, different bureaucrats value life differently.[12] The United States Department of Transport puts a price of $1 million on a human life. The Consumer Product Safety Commission values that life at $2 million, while the Environmental Protection Agency (EPA) has a sliding scale of $450,000 to $8 million.

A human price tag makes life easier for bureaucrats. EPA in 1984 proposed a draft regulation banning asbestos, a well-known human cancer agent. (By this date large numbers of Second World War shipyard workers who had worked with asbestos had already died.) The asbestos industry lobbied successfully to have the Office of Management and Budget (OMB) block the proposal. OMB defended their decision on the basis of cost to the industry and asbestos consumers versus cost of human lives that would be lost to cancer. The OMB bureaucrats started out in their cost/benefit calculation by valuing a human life at $1 million, but then they discounted the value. They said that the asbestos-caused cancer only occurs many years after exposure, and therefore, the dead cancer victim actually misses fewer years of a natural lifespan. So they discounted his value to $208,000. As *Time* put it, 'at such bargain prices, the regulation wasn't cost efficient.'[13]

The Real Environment

Risk assessment is a bureaucratic way of looking at the world. I mentioned earlier the controversy over Alar (daminozide), a chemical sprayed on apples to strengthen their stems. At question was the interpretation of Alar's risk assessment: the EPA and Uniroyal Chemical Company, the maker, felt that the amount of Alar in apples was below the threshold at which it causes harm; the public, especially parents of children, felt otherwise. Uniroyal withdrew the product when apple sales plummeted. But throughout the controversy the fact that apples are contaminated with the residues of two dozen or more pesticides, plus an unknown number of industrial chemicals, did not enter public debate, although apple eaters and cider drinkers are exposed to the whole cocktail. Risk assessment based on Alar failed to address this cocktail. The combinations of different pesticides and industrial chemicals vary from apple to apple, so there is no way of knowing what is on your particular apple. Government regulators say that because of this uncertainty they do not know how to assess the cocktail. Thus the real hazard of eating apples remains unknown, even unstudied.

Environment bureaucrats, because they say they have no alternative, stick with risk assessment of single chemicals. This perseverance amounts to an addiction, and like other forms of addiction, it gives a false sense of safety; and, critically, it removes the incentive to come up with an alternative that would give a more realistic appraisal of the world.

Risk assessment is intended to give a number that tells whether or not the chemical is safe; bureaucrats like it because they can make a decision based on a number. But when they have to deal with the real world of multiple chemicals their decision-making breaks down. This is what happened to the Canadian government, faced with chemical pollution in the Arctic, home of some 22,000 Eskimos.[14] Scientists found an alarming degree of contamination by industrial chemicals in Eskimo foods and in the Eskimos themselves. An assortment of persistent pesticides, like DDT and Lindane, PCBs, dioxins and dozens of other noxious chemicals are carried northwards by air and sea currents where they enter the Arctic food chain. The Arctic acts like a giant sink.

Barry Hargrave, a marine ecologist working in the Arctic, said that another reason why the Eskimos are at greater risk is that so much of their food is animal. They are at the top of the Arctic food chain, and their diet of seal, walrus, beluga whales and fish is contaminated. Arctic animals tend to store a lot of fat and that is where the chemical contaminants lodge. The Eskimos eat all that fat, accumulating the contaminants in their own body fat.[15]

It is not hard to analyse human fat samples and samples from marine animals and plant life for all these noxious chemicals. That part of the science is easy. What is hard is trying to interpret this information in terms of the lives of real people. The human population is by no means uniformly resistant to the effects of the pollution: some are young; some are old; some are pregnant and some are weakened by illness. How the toxic harm will manifest itself and in how many individuals is completely unknown.

The Arctic situation is like a patient coming into a doctor's surgery with a vague complaint that defies diagnosis. The doctor is unable to do much. Likewise, the Canadian government, unable to carry out a risk assessment, was left up the proverbial creek without a paddle. So they did nothing. They really had no precedent or means to assess the Arctic situation and officials were left making non-scientific, speculative statements. David Kinloch, a medical officer in the region, said 'It's very worrisome because so much of the population [of the Arctic region] depends on country foods.'[16] He defined country foods as wild game, and added that the inhabitants do not dilute their food intake by eating other foods, as southern people do.

The Eskimos cannot wall their Arctic environment off from the industrial world, so their only recourse may be to eat expensive frozen turkey and canned spaghetti flown in at great cost from southern Canada. (A 10 kg turkey costs $70 in the Canadian north.) It is not a solution that the Brundtland Commission would be likely to admire.

Risk Assessment Fails to Give an Ecological Perspective

There is another aspect of risk assessment that goes beyond the pure science: the frame of mind it engenders. I cited above the example of the Canadian Arctic to show how risk assessment, which can only be applied to single chemicals, is of no value in arriving at a policy decision; but the idea of assessing risk is still there. In other words, the government speculated in general about the health risk of living in the Canadian Arctic. Risk assessment encourages thinking about such problems in isolation rather than looking at the broader environmental issue, which, in this case, is movement of toxic chemicals into that environment from the industrial south. The only solution is to deal with the chemicals at their source.

But there is great reluctance to think in broader terms. One source of the Eskimos' contamination is the pulp and paper industry. North

American paper mills bleach the pulp used in making toilet tissue with chlorine or chlorine dioxide. This bleaching agent, similar to household bleach, changes the dull brown of the pulp to a pure white, but the agent reacts with substances in the pulp producing trace amounts of chlorinated chemicals (organochlorines) by the dozen, including dioxins. Dioxin and other contaminants of the toilet tissue can cause cancer and a host of other ills, and they are absorbed easily through the skin with every swipe at your bottom. And from the Eskimos' perspective, the mills discharge enormous quantities of contaminated waste water into the nearest water body. The organochlorines evaporate from the warmer waters where the mills are located and are carried northward by prevailing winds where they accumulate in the cold water of the Arctic region.

The presence of the toxic organochlorines in bleached pulp has been known to United States and Canadian governments for many years, but the only response has been inaction. The Swedish government outlawed chlorine bleaching several years ago, and Swedish pulp mills switched either to hydrogen peroxide bleaching (which does not produce the chemicals) or, for some products, no bleach at all. Swedish consumers seem happy with the tan-coloured products, knowing they are free of the toxic organochlorines.

Public outrage has been less strong in North America, which is one reason why pulp mills have not dropped chlorine bleach, according to Bill McKloy of the Council of British Columbia Forest Industries. He said the Canadian consumer will have to show there is a strong demand for products free of organochlorines. (The plight of the Eskimos did not enter into this discussion.) He gave another reason for not changing: cost. The capital costs of switching to a chlorine-free bleach could run to $40 million for a pulp mill.[17] Canadian and United States government officials say they are maintaining a 'watching brief' on the situation.

One fallout of thinking of environmental problems in isolation is a failure to link chemical pollution of the Arctic with white toilet paper, or with Alar, or with other pesticides, and so on. Government policy-makers would rather make a risk assessment of each chemical and deal with the public one chemical at a time, and as a result government officials tend to stagger from issue to issue: today it's Alar; tomorrow it's some other pesticide or an industrial dump. It is a dog's perspective of a forest, a dash from tree to tree, a quick lift of the leg at each. There is a failure to develop an overview of environmental issues and develop comprehensive policies that prevent the environmental hazards from arising.

Risk assessment is a direct cause-and-effect exercise: it disallows the taking of a broad ecological view of the human environment and all its connections. I started this chapter by commenting how the health-care system influences environmental policy, and we see here what happens when a medical tool is applied to the environment as a basis for decision-making. The medical doctors have a point – you have to identify a problem before you can take effective action; but risk assessment is hardly the way to identify environmental problems.

7

Ecotoxicity

'We knew the groundwater on our farm was bad, so for two years we drank the town water, just to be safe.' Steve Shivvers had been bringing plastic bottles of town water to his farm 10 km out of Corydon, a small town of 1,800 population in southern Iowa, when he learned that the town's tap water was also contaminated. 'Now what are we supposed to do?' he said in interview with a *New York Times* reporter.[1]

Shivvers must have felt like a goldfish in a bowl of contaminated water: he couldn't stop using water. There was no place to turn; his farm well and the town water were both contaminated, and there was no other source of water in his area. Shivvers's well, like half the farm wells in Iowa, was contaminated with toxic pesticide residues, so Shivvers started using the town water which came from a surface reservoir. But State researchers in the spring of 1987 found Corydon's tap water contaminated with pesticides and fertilizers that had washed into the town's reservoir ·with the spring rains. The town's water purification plant did not remove the chemicals. Shivvers's environment had turned toxic, not toxic in the sense that he, his wife Diane and their two children were ill, but toxic in terms of a threat to their long-term family well-being.

Environmental toxicity, or ecotoxicity as it is sometimes called, is a new form of toxic hazard that threatens not only farm people but everyone on the globe. There is a sense of being trapped. It is not the usual kind of toxicity, where you are poisoned by a single dose of, say, arsenic, that can sicken you with deadly quickness. You can avoid the toxicity of arsenic by avoiding arsenic, but you cannot avoid ecotoxicity because it affects your drinking water, food and every breath of air. The amounts of poisons are low, but your exposure grinds on day after day, year after year. It is your environment that is toxic.

Ecotoxicity results from chemicals that enter the environment from waste sites, municipal sewers and industrial leakage, or, as in the case of farm chemicals, are deliberately applied to the environment. Once there, the chemicals cycle through land, air and water; the environment cannot be purified, and the best you can hope for is the gradual breakdown of the chemicals. But chemicals continually leak into the environment, so contamination is an ongoing factor of modern life.

Ecotoxicity is like being eaten by a thousand ants. It takes a while, but eventually the bites wear you down. It is poisoning in slow motion. Whereas scientists have a good idea of the fast motion effects of a dose of a single chemical like arsenic, their knowledge of what long-term exposure to environmental chemicals does to you is imprecise. Scientists do know, however, that when large populations are exposed over a long period to low levels of toxic chemicals, a certain percentage of the population contracts a variety of illnesses, from cancer to ill-defined aches and pains and unsettling neurological disorders. But medical scientists are unable to predict which members of the exposed population will be made ill or in what way they will be made ill.

It is not surprising, given such vagueness and imprecision, that scientists are unable to put numbers on the problem. Their methods of risk assessment are all but useless. Ecotoxicity is something that has crept up on the world population over the last twenty-five years, and the scientific and medical communities have not really figured out how to study the problem, let alone assess it. What is happening now is a growing recognition that there is a problem, but what the problem is and what to do about it remain, to say the least, vague.

Single Chemical Assessment of Ecotoxicity

It is this uncertainty that faced Darrell McAllister, chief of the Surface and Groundwater Protection Office of the Iowa Department of Natural Resources when his office found traces of pesticides and fertilizers in the drinking water of Corydon and thirty other Iowa towns. His problem was trying to interpret the findings to Iowa citizens. The EPA, with its large laboratories and financial resources, was supposed to be establishing national drinking water standards, but after eighteen years of study this project was barely off the drawing board. Iowa farmers use over 200 different pesticides, and McAllister had analysed the water samples for residues of thirty-seven of these pesticides. But for only one of the thirty-seven, the herbicide 2,4-D (2,4-dichlorophenoxyacetic acid), was there an EPA standard under the Safe Drinking Water Act. In addition, EPA had set preliminary standards, what it called advisory levels, for two more of the pesticides on McAllister's list, Atrazine and Metalachlor. The EPA was thus able to give McAllister three standards from a pool of 200 commonly used pesticides.

At this point, there is a need to spell out the difference between ecotoxicity as it exists and ecotoxicity as it is perceived by the EPA, and for that matter by all environmental agencies of industrialized countries. True ecotoxicity is that of Eskimos and goldfish: total exposure to everything – food, air, water – in one's environment. The body has to detoxify this total burden. But the EPA, in the interests of bureaucratic regulation, ignores total exposure and performs a risk assessment of each toxic chemical as if all other contaminating chemicals were absent. It is a deceptive task, because to assess such a threat precisely it would be necessary to find people living in a pristine environment and then expose them to the one chemical for which they wish to specify a standard. There is no pristine environment left anywhere in the world; every human on the globe is exposed to a multiplicity of chemical contaminants.

The EPA approach to ecotoxicity is like that of an entomologist who assesses the thousand ants eating you by issuing standards on the bites of three of them, saying be careful of these three. So here is how the EPA's approach to assessment of water safety worked for McAllister, based on the two preliminary standards for Atrazine and Metalachlor. It set what it calls a lifetime health advisory level of 2.5 parts per billion (ppb) for Atrazine and 10.5 ppb for Metalachlor. EPA officials estimate that these levels (not yet written into law) represent the maximum exposure an individual can tolerate over a lifetime without appreciable health risk. (The standards are in fact vague guesses based on laboratory work with animals.)

During the spring runoff the amounts of the two pesticides in Corydon's tap water exceeded the EPA's advisory level, but at other times of the year water analysis showed 0.9 ppb for Atrazine and 0.33 ppb for Metalachlor, well below the EPA's maximum levels. If you accepted the EPA's method of assessing ecotoxicity and you were McAllister telling the residents what to do, you might say: 'Don't drink the water during spring runoff, but it is safe the rest of the year.'

McAllister was not reassured by EPA's criteria of safety which gave a green light to the water for summer, autumn and winter. These criteria left unanswered such questions as: What about all the other pesticide residues that weren't analysed? What about the fact that Corydon's water is permanently contaminated with Atrazine and Metalachlor? How can the EPA be sure that levels of 0.9 and 0.33 ppb over an Iowan's lifetime are not harmful? McAllister was worried. 'It shows we don't know how often these kinds of results are going to be seen or how sustained they are,' he said in interview. 'That's what is so scary about this.'[2]

It is no secret why Iowa's water is contaminated. Iowa farmers use 34 million kg (75 million lb) of pesticides in a growing season, 11 kg (25 lb) for every inhabitant of the state, two tons per square kilometre of land. Some of that tonnage breaks down, some is washed into the surface water of streams and some percolates into the groundwater. The pesticides include insecticides and fungicides, but over half of the tonnage is weedkillers – herbicides.

In addition to the pesticides, Iowa farmers use vast quantities of fertilizer. American farmers as a whole apply about 50 million metric tons (45 million tons) per year. Farmers heap it on hoping to squeeze out yields that extra bit higher, but it is far more than the plants can use: as much as half of it percolates into the water table. The result is that groundwater becomes a soup of various chemicals, and the three quarters of the Iowan population that gets its drinking water from the ground drinks the entire soup.[3]

Is Ecotoxicity a Health Threat?

This chemical soup has no official existence. The EPA confines its assessment of groundwater safety to the standards of the three pesticides. To get an inkling of the effects of drinking the chemical soup, we have to turn to epidemiological evidence, and that is only sketchy at best.

Iowa officials found a sharp increase in certain cancers among farmers compared with residents in other parts of the United States, and noted that this increase paralleled the increase in use of pesticides over the last three decades. (The studies did not pinpoint any particular pesticide.) Cancer is one of the easiest effects of ecotoxicity to pick up in a study because the statistics are generally well recorded. The Iowa study was done by obtaining the data from the registrar of deaths, then comparing the incidence of cancer in Iowa with the incidence in a similar population in a non-farming region. Because cancer studies are relatively easy to do and because cancer has a neon-light profile, cancer risk becomes the indicator for the presence or absence of ecotoxicity: officials often state that because the cancer risk is low in a certain situation, there is no ecotoxicity to worry about.

It would be nice if the real world operated so simply, but it does not. Exposure to environmental chemicals can dislocate the workings of the human body in many ways. We have a general idea about such damage, but exact effects are less easy to pinpoint and the records of such effects are poorly kept. The result is that we have to rely on scraps of information that come to light. Here, as an example, is one such scrap.

The reproductive organs contain some of the body's most intricate biochemical mechanisms, and we know that contaminating chemicals can act like grit in a watch. Health officials in California found a higher than average number of miscarriages and babies born with birth defects among women who drank groundwater, polluted (in this case) by chemical solvents, than among a group of women who drank city water thought to be uncontaminated.[4] The surprise in the study came when they looked at a third group of women who drank bottled water. This group had even fewer miscarriages and about half the number of babies with birth defects than among the city tap-water drinkers.

The worrisome implication of this unexpected finding is that municipal water that has gone through treatment plants before it gets to householders' taps contains a level of contaminants sufficient to raise the number of birth defects. And if this is true in the California district, is it true everywhere, because chemical contamination is everywhere? In other words, the background level of contamination is increasing and because everyone is affected the rise is not so obvious. You do not notice the rise unless you compare two groups, one more seriously affected than the other. Health officials thus come to accept as the norm a level of miscarriages and birth defects which may in fact be elevated above what need be the case.

Teratogenicity is a word derived from the Greek which means monster-causing; it is one of the outcomes of chemical exposure. In simpler language, teratogenicity means birth defects and miscarriages. Chemicals that are teratogenic act on the fetus at some point in the first seven months of pregnancy, disrupting its orderly development and causing a permanent defect, which may be serious enough to arrest fetal development; the fetus then spontaneously aborts in a miscarriage.

Not all chemicals are teratogenic, but a group of experts in human reproduction sponsored by the American Medical Association noted that many chemicals (including pesticides) commonly found in people's home environment – in their food, drinking water and air – are teratogenic.[5] This study, however, was based on feeding the chemicals individually to pregnant laboratory animals and looking for teratogenic effects. The scientists did not look at the kinds of mixtures of chemicals to which women are exposed, nor at what the risk is when exposure is at low levels.

Nevertheless, a message emerges from all these studies: long-term exposure to a variety of chemicals at low levels can measurably increase the risk of harm to the human reproductive systems: not just to females and their developing fetuses, but to males also, because exposure of males to chemicals may affect the sperm in such a way that there is increased risk of fathering a defective child.

This kind of information does not enter the mindset of the EPA because birth defects and miscarriages are not connected to any chemical on the EPA's list of standards. EPA officials will say the information is too woolly; 'we can't use it in setting standards for chemical contaminants in drinking water.' And they are right; but only because they think in terms of standardizing single chemicals. If they thought in terms of ecotoxicity, that is, in terms of the total situation – the water itself – they would be able to see that it is the water and all its contents that is toxic.

What is the US Government doing to Protect Groundwater?

The US Congress, frustrated at the EPA's grinding pace in setting standards for chemical contaminants of groundwater (in addition to the three pesticides, it has set standards for thirty-five other substances out of a potential of 100,000 industrial chemicals), has frequently tried to light fires under the EPA to hurry it along. But Congress never questions whether the standard-setting approach was the most effective way of tackling groundwater contamination. The EPA's approach to ecotoxicity – the setting of standards for selected chemicals – was set into law by Congress. But curiously, while Congress gave the EPA the task of standard-setting, it gave it little clout to do anything about violations of the standards. This fact does not seem to bother EPA officials, and one finds an almost childlike faith that once the standards are set (several centuries from now, at the current rate, in spite of Congress's prodding) assessment of water safety will be easy. This dislocation between assessment and enforcement becomes apparent in the case of contaminated groundwater. How, for example, does one provide pesticide- and fertilizer-free water to the citizens of Corydon, or any other community dependent on groundwater? Marion Mlay, director of the EPA's groundwater programme, when questioned about action, said that the EPA could try to restrict application of agricultural chemicals though labelling, but conceded, 'enforcement is difficult. EPA depends on the good senses of people applying it.'[6]

What of the good sense of the agriculturalists, the people applying the chemicals? William Storck, an editor of *Chemical and Engineering News*, surveyed journals published by the United States Department of Agriculture (USDA). The department's concern was limited. Its official journal, *Agricultural Outlook*, has published articles outlining methods to prevent farm chemicals from polluting coastal waters. But the main concern of USDA is economic: the waste of expensive pesticides and fertilizers. *Agricultural Resources*, another USDA publication, contained an article in its August 1987 issue which had little to say about contaminated water, being more concerned with an aroused public that might demand a ban on certain pesticides. If Atrazine were banned, the article said, corn yields would drop an estimated 8 per cent and its price would rise by 31 per cent.[7]

USDA does not have what one might term a broad outlook, but its position too is a reflection of government attitudes. In an attempt to expand its horizon on the groundwater problem, the House of Representatives in 1987 passed the Groundwater Research Act with the idea of funding a study of contamination from farm chemicals. The legislators believed that what was needed was a base line of the current level of contamination in order to measure future contamination. The Act, in recognition that the agricultural sector is a major source of the contamination, established an Agriculture Task Force to find ways to reduce groundwater contamination from fertilizer use.

But legislators, in deference to heavy lobbying from the agricultural chemical industry and farm organizations, excluded pesticides from the Task Force's charge, although pesticides are probably a greater contributor to groundwater ecotoxicity than fertilizer.[8] Were the industry and farm groups afraid of the information the Task Force would turn up? In any event, the Act fosters talk, not action. The sources of groundwater contamination are known; what are lacking are policy decisions to prevent contamination from occurring.

Groundwater Contamination is a Problem in Britain

The political quandary over what to do about contaminated groundwater is not restricted to the United States. Thirty-five per cent of the tap water of England and Wales comes from underground aquifers. Water authority officials insist the water is 'safe and wholesome', but when you probe into what they know about the water, this turns out to be very little. The only chemicals in tap water to which the government applies standards are nitrates (from fertilizers).[9] Yet when tap water is checked, the whole range of industrial and agricultural chemicals can show up. One study by scientists of Imperial College, London found significant contamination by chemical solvents of 40 per cent of wells checked.

Britain is particularly vulnerable to groundwater contamination. Forty-six million people and their industries and farms occupy an area the size of Iowa. A lot of the underlying geology of the country is porous chalk, and surface water and contaminants rapidly penetrate into the aquifers. Mike Price, a hydrogeologist of the British Geological Survey, calculated that as little as 5 tons of certain highly toxic chemicals would be enough to contaminate one year's rainfall for the entire chalk outcrops.

The social situation in Britain is similar to that in the United States: the general public has a feeling of widespread and insidious ecotoxicity connected with groundwater, but no clear understanding of it. The government is unable to provide enlightenment. With chemical monitoring limited to nitrates, the government has no firm grasp of the health effects of the total chemical soup and is able to foster an illusion that ecotoxicity does not exist.

The government's main efforts, in fact, have been in public relations, downplaying the importance of the contamination. Critics say that its main concern is to satisfy a legal mandate of the European Economic Community (EEC) rather than to deal with threats to the public's health. They note that Britain lags considerably behind its European partners in addressing the problem of contaminated water. The EEC has set safety limits for fifty chemicals in drinking water, and if these limits are exceeded Britain could be sued in the European court.

But again, this is arguing over standards. Standards do not reflect the ecotoxicity of European groundwater any more than that of groundwater in the United States. On both continents, the water is contaminated with an undetermined mix of toxic chemicals. The governments' picture of the groundwater situation is like a child's drawing of its mother; it is indeed a picture of sorts, but it is not a picture the police would use for identification. Standard-setting fails to give us a useful picture of ecotoxicity and all its ramifications for human health and for the ecosystem.

Silent Autumn

One of the problems with trying to address environmental contamination with individual standards is that just having standards does not indicate what to do. Having standards for a handful of chemicals in no way matches the environmental reality of a toxic soup consisting of tens of thousands of different chemicals trickling twenty-four hours every day from many sources: toxic waste dumps, municipal garbage, wanton disposal of chemicals, agricultural chemicals.

In order to indicate the complexity of the problem and what bureaucrats are doing or not doing about it, I have concentrated on one sector: farm chemicals and groundwater. But as the argument over the use of farm chemicals unfolds, the whole dilemma over chemical contamination of the environment is revealed. The argument is generally couched in terms of benefit versus risk – the solid economic benefits of high crop yields versus the vague health risks of ecotoxicity. Recognizing the danger of over-simplifying the different positions among the public on this argument, let us nevertheless say that there are two poles: one pole says you cannot farm without chemicals so therefore one has to put up with the toxic risks; the other pole says the risks are too great and besides, you can indeed farm without chemicals, so why use them? The contrast could be stated another way: for example, with chemical pesticides, one pole of the argument looks upon pesticides as magic bullets going straight to their targets and doing their job; the other pole sees the pesticides acting like a shotgun hitting everything indiscriminately.

Dow Chemical Company, Midland, Michigan, a major manufacturer of pesticides and a proponent of the magic bullet argument, published a booklet, entitled *Silent Autumn*. The title is an obvious takeoff of Rachel Carson's 1962 book, *Silent Spring*, which predicted ecological devastation from continued use of pesticides. *Silent Autumn* predicts what would come about if Rachel Carson's successors had their way and banned farm chemicals.

The Dow Company's position is akin to that of drug companies that without drugs there can be no health: without farm chemicals there can be no harvests. Dow has allies in government departments of agriculture which are also firm followers of this dictum. Perhaps one of the dictum's most expressive publicists was Earl Butz, formerly dean of the School of Agriculture at Purdue University and US Secretary of Agriculture during the Nixon and Ford presidencies. If we give up pesticides and other technologies of modern agriculture, Butz would say, we have to ask which 50 million Americans we are going to let starve. Butz's message was clear: without pesticides, production of food would not support the present American population.

Butz's argument may seem extreme, but what he said was true to the extent that crop production would plummet if farmers gave up pesticides. People would be eating a lot of insect-infested fruits and vegetables. The reason is that chemical pesticides are built into the modern practice of farming; you could say that they, in fact, are its foundation. What Butz is saying is, take away the foundation and modern farming would collapse. But he and other champions of chemical-intensive agriculture assume that the only way to farm is horizon-to-horizon single crops. The State of Iowa is seeded almost entirely to soybeans and corn, the same crop being planted in the same fields year after year – a monocrop. Insects and weeds love monocrops: the same conditions are repeated each growing season, attracting pest species galore.

The monocrop is defenceless without its pesticides, but pesticides do not eradicate weeds or insects; they simply hold populations in check. Without pesticides, the weed and insect populations literally explode. So Butz has a point: take pesticides away from the current generation of monocropping farmers and you leave them stark naked in a cloud of insects and weed pollen.

No wonder agricultural officials look upon advocates of a switch to non-chemical farming as cranks and oddballs. Modern farming is organized around monocropping, and farmers will specialize in one or at most two crops, honing their skills to produce just those crops. Farmers are also businessmen, and they invest heavily in the specialized equipment designed to produce that crop: and which is useless for handling other crops. Moreover, the farmer becomes plugged into an infrastructure of seed and chemical suppliers and buyers of his speciality crops. All this would have to be adjusted if farmers gave up pesticides. But the adjustment is not as difficult as advocates of chemical-intensive farming would have us believe and the payoffs in pesticide-free crops and groundwater would be enormous. We will come to the alternative, non-chemical farming in a moment, but let us continue for now with commentary on the downside of chemical pesticides.

Pesticides are not Magic Bullets

A compelling reason, besides the withdrawal symptoms, why agricultural officials shrug off critics of pesticides is that they believe pesticides as used in the field are safe, and this belief persists in spite of a growing body of evidence to the contrary. Agriculturalists remain firm believers in the magic bullet.

When Paul Ehrlich at the turn of the century conceived his idea of a magic bullet for treating human illness, he set the conceptual stage for pesticides as well – the idea that a chemical would selectively seek out a weed or insect and kill it without harm to the crop. Ehrlich's discovery of the anti-syphilis drug Salvarsan had a profound effect on agriculturalists. Could magic bullets be devised that selectively destroy pests? Forty years passed after Ehrlich's Salvarsan emerged before the first magic pesticide was discovered: DDT.

DDT indeed seemed at first glance the perfect magic bullet. Marketed in the closing phases of the Second World War, it prevented typhus from spreading among troops and civilian populations. Typhus, a deadly infection, is spread by body lice, and most people in the battle areas harboured lice because of the abominable sanitary conditions. Exterminators poured DDT on the heads and down the pants of everyone they could find. The lice were exterminated, their human hosts apparently unaffected by the pesticide.

DDT was used extensively in European and North American agriculture until about 1970, when it was banned. People had realized by this time that it was a bullet without magic. What happened? Nothing predictable from laboratory experiments. Wildlife biologists began to report a crash in the populations of peregrine falcons, seagulls and other birds, which they traced to thin eggshells. The adult birds seemed healthy enough, flying about and catching fish, but their eggshells were so thin the eggs cracked from the weight of the sitting bird. Biologists determined that the female bird's oviduct failed to put down an adequate amount of calcium. The cause: DDT.

DDT is a splendid pesticide because it is virtually indestructible. That was considered a virtue when DDT was first introduced, but as the tonnage of DDT applied each year simply added to the tonnage of previous years, more and more accumulated in the environment. Moreover, DDT is volatile, which means that it evaporates into the atmosphere and is carried to other parts of the world where it is washed to the earth's surface by rain. (DDT is one of the contaminating chemicals of the Arctic.) It was soon possible to detect DDT in the body fat of Arctic seals, polar bears and beluga whales.

In the sea world of the peregrine falcon, DDT accumulates in plankton, which is eaten by tiny sea creatures, which in turn are eaten by larger creatures, the DDT passing from creature to creature until it reaches the falcon at the top of the food chain. Each plant or animal in the chain accumulates the DDT, concentrating it as much as a million times. By the time DDT gets to the falcon the concentration is high enough to wreck the female's oviduct.

It is this ability of all organisms, including humans, to suck up chemical contaminants like vacuum cleaners and concentrate them in body tissues that makes predictions of ecotoxicity so difficult. The amount of DDT in drinking water is infinitesimal and if that amount were the criterion of safety one could say it was insignificant. But DDT bioaccumulates in body tissues, and today, twenty years after it was banned, DDT is still present in substantial amounts in human milk. The risk is now passed on to babies. It is the sort of risk that somehow does not get included in the benefit/risk ratio of using farm chemicals.

DDT is only one of dozens of environmental chemicals in mothers' milk. All women in North America and Europe have accumulated these chemicals from the time of their own birth until twenty to thirty years later when they have a child. The mother's body literally drains the chemicals, first into the fetus during pregnancy, then into the milk, and as much as a third of her body burden can pass into the baby, one fifteenth her own size. Does any harm to the child result? Studies carried out by a team headed by Walter Rogan and sponsored by the National Institute of Environmental Health, North Carolina, showed a retardation in babies' development.[10] The team first studied babies born to Taiwanese mothers who had been accidentally exposed to polychlorinated biphenyls (PCBs). Their babies were born smaller and had a variety of physical defects ranging from presence of teeth to the acne more commonly seen in teenagers. They followed up with a second study on mothers and their babies in North Carolina. In this case, there was no known special contamination, just the chemical background of all citizens. The mothers' bodies contained PCBs and dozens of other chemicals including farm pesticides; some had more, some had less. Rogan's team found that the higher the body burden of the mother the less well the baby was able to co-ordinate muscular movements – apparently an effect on the developing nervous system. Their data suggest that the main effect is during the fetal stage when the fetus is much smaller and the nervous system is developing. The additional amount of chemicals received from the milk after birth did not affect their co-ordination.

Again, as with the California study of birth defects and exposure to tap water, these studies indicate that the low level of chemical contamination is sufficient to damage human biology. It is important to note that this impairment in development can be picked up only through special studies; it is not something a doctor examining a baby in his surgery would notice. The health effect in this case is subclinical, yet by and large it is such subclinical effects that ecotoxicity produces. Note also that the parents suffer no obvious effects; it is the developing fetus and infant that is vulnerable.

This kind of information gives environmental bureaucrats a big head-ache, for two reasons. First, they regulate chemical contaminants on the basis that the chemical might cause some overt clinical disease to adults, like cancer or liver disease. Here the mother is contaminated over years with no apparent harm, the ultimate harm being passed on to the next generation. Second, they have no bureaucratic mechanism for regulating chemical soups; their procedures deal with single chemicals. Moreover, to regulate, the bureaucrats have to identify specific sources. Trying to identify specific sources of the chemical soup in mother's milk would be like being shot at by a shotgun and trying to identify which particular pellet or pellets hit their mark. The single-chemical approach to controlling chemical contamination of the environment is not capable of dealing with the real world of toxic soups. The only solution to contaminated wombs is to prevent the contamination from occurring in the first place.

The Cañete: an Answer to Chemical Pesticides

How would you prevent the contamination of the womb and mother's milk? You have to go to the sources of contamination, each and every one of them. To illustrate the preventive approach with respect to one source, I come back to farms and their chemicals. Champions of chemical farming would immediately object to making any link between their practices and infant feeding. They can point out that the milk contains industrial chemicals as well as pesticide and fertilizer residues, and that therefore the farm sector cannot be blamed for the soup. This immediate response, of course, is cause-and-effect thinking; unless a specific pesticide residue can be linked to specific effects on infants then nothing should be done. Such thinking provokes endless argument and no action. The residues farm chemicals leave are part of the environmental chemical soup, and instead of worrying what chemical does what, why not clean up the agricultural chemicals as a group? The idea is not to ban pesticides overnight – Silent Autumn could be the result – but to shift the method of farming so that it phases out the need for pesticides and ensures agricultural production.

That this can be done is illustrated by the story of one farming community, that of the Cañete Valley of Peru, about 120 km (72 miles) south-east of Lima. The valley is a self-contained agricultural system growing mostly cotton. For decades, until the 1940s, growers controlled insect pests by simple means. They continually inspected their crops and counted the number of insects in each field, a technique that gave them a population history of the insects, enabling them to predict accurately when the population was about to surge. They would then spray with slow-acting, short-lived, mild insecticides. Beneficial insects were not harmed, and in this way, the farmers maintained good control over pest populations.[11]

But, like a cat which leaps into an easy chair when given the chance, the Cañete growers in the 1940s adopted DDT, benzene hexachloride and toxaphene when they came on the market. These seeming magic bullets wiped out all the insects. Yields soared. The growers were elated; but their elation was short-lived. In less than ten years the old pests had developed resistance to the three pesticides, and new insect pests appeared that no one had ever noticed before. In 1956 the growers lost 70 per cent of their cotton.

The chemical companies told the growers: 'use heavier doses more frequently' and 'buy the newer pesticides that we have.' But the Peruvian government, sceptical of these claims, refused to allow the growers to buy the new chemicals and instead recommended changes in growing practices that encouraged natural predators of the insect pests. Damage decreased, yields jumped once more, and for the last thirty years cotton production has remained higher than it ever was in the heyday of chemical pesticides.

Chemical pesticides repelled the Peruvian authorities for two reasons: they were uneasy about potential health hazards to the residents in the Cañete Valley, and they found that pesticides did not do the job the chemical companies said they would. This government rejection of chemical pesticides, however, is rare; on a worldwide basis, application of pesticides of all types has multiplied many times over the last thirty years and continues to rise.

So we have a paradox: a world agriculture increasingly dependent on a technology of pest control that does not work all that well, and a world population that is asked to accept the ecotoxicity that goes with chemical pesticide use because chemical pesticides are deemed irreplaceable.

Are they really irreplaceable? The farmers of the Cañete manage without them, but agriculturists argue that the Cañete is an isolated, small valley and that the non-chemical controls they use would not work on the broad scale of agriculture in North America and Europe. Nevertheless, an undercurrent of disquiet about the extensive use of pesticide technology runs through farming circles in northern countries.

This disquiet surfaces in the search for alternative, non-chemical ways of farming.

Biological Farming

The agricultural system of the United States has firmly embraced the tradition of Earl Butz, so it seemed out of character when in the late 1970s the then Secretary of Agriculture, Robert Bergland, commissioned a survey of organic farmers. The definition of 'organic' is that the farmer avoids use of chemical fertilizers and pesticides, favouring instead crop rotation, cultivation, composting and other strategies to ensure crop yield. Such techniques also go under the name of biological, biodynamic or ecological farming.

Bergland's survey turned up 30,000 US farmers who fell into this category. Contrary to expectations that most such farmers would be farming at a subsistence level, the survey found them to be prosperous. Their yields were sometimes lower than those of the chemical-intensive farmer, but as they did not have to buy the expensive pesticides and fertilizers, and their net profit – determined by price received for crops less cost of inputs – was excellent. This is a simple lesson that many chemical-intensive farmers seem to ignore in their single-minded goal of maximizing yield; they forget the high cost of their chemical inputs.

The organic farmers, when asked why they farmed that way, gave several reasons: they were afraid of being poisoned by the pesticides; their profits were greater; they felt that chemical-intensive farming was somehow not in accord with nature.

USDA disowned the Bergland report on the change of administration in 1980, and the organic farmers were left on their own. USDA research stations concentrated all their efforts on making chemical-intensive agriculture even more intensive. But some ten years later, interest in organic farming in political circles has reawakened. One reason for this reawakening is a change in name. The term 'organic' did not sit well in official agriculture. It smacked of a back-to-nature movement, not at all in keeping with the macho image of conquering nature with chemicals. The new term is 'sustainable agriculture', a term that somehow seems less threatening.

'This kind of research [sustainable] could eventually bring about the healthiest agriculture in the world,' said Senator Patrick Leahy, Chairman of the Senate Agriculture Committee. Leahy was responding to the creation in 1987 of the country's first chair for studying sustainable farm practices at the University of Minnesota.[12] The university research, according to Leahy, will help wean Minnesota farmers from their chemical dependency, and promote farming practices that avoid degradation of soil and water.

Ken Tschumper is one Minnesota farmer already proving that sustainable agriculture works. He stopped using chemicals six years ago on his dairy farm in La Crescent and switched to non-chemical control of insects and to crop rotation: corn, oats and alfalfa. The oats crowd out weeds, preventing them from reseeding, and the alfalfa, a legume, adds nitrogen to the soil which benefits the corn next season. Neighbours initially ridiculed Tschumper, saying he would soon be bankrupt; instead, his farm flourished. He says that he can produce a bushel of corn for 40 cents, compared to $2.00 for his chemical neighbours. He added $20,000 to his savings account in 1987, while several of his neighbours, hit by low corn prices, filed for bankruptcy. Tschumper said, 'when you don't use chemicals, you become a much better observer [of nature] – you're constantly evaluating conditions. It verges on the artistic.'[13]

Government policy, however, backs chemical farming and farmers like Tschumper receive little technical backup from the government. The same paradox holds in European countries. One thousand British farmers, for example, scattered all over the country, farm organically and profitably. They and similar farmers in other European countries are unable to meet public demand for organically grown crops, which suggests that British consumers like the idea of buying food grown under chemical-free conditions. A National Opinion Poll conducted in Britain in 1988, in fact, found that 60 per cent of consumers wish that farmers would avoid the use of chemicals.

This wish is not shared by the British government, which provides no support for chemical-free farming. The government has a policy of maximizing production (in spite of mountainous agricultural surpluses) and a policy of supporting chemical farming as the instrument to achieve that maximum. The government pursues its policy of chemical agriculture in spite of evidence that the chemicals are polluting groundwater and in spite of evidence that chemicals are unnecessary. The Elm Tree Research Centre, Newbury, Berkshire, a champion of organic agriculture, claims that farmers could make chemical-free farming the mainstream option for British agriculture and still sustain government production goals.[14]

One does not have to be a genius to recognize the economic pressures in this debate over chemical versus non-chemical farming. If the farmers of North America and Europe go the route of Ken Tschumper, agricultural chemicals go the route of the steam locomotive. Chemical companies are sensitive to complaints about the pollution that their products cause and to the fact that the effectiveness of many pesticides is slipping; they say privately, 'we'll milk the chemical pesticides as long as we can, but what we have in the laboratory will secure our financial security.' What they have up their laboratory sleeve is genetically engineered plants and animals.

This new agricultural technology introduces plants and animals created in the laboratory that offer features considered important in chemical-intensive agriculture: greater yield, insect resistance, greater size. Chemical companies say the new techniques reduce the need for the kinds of chemical pesticides now on the market. But there is no guarantee that bio-engineered corn plants and cows will not introduce some new, unanticipated set of environmental problems. The farming practices of Ken Tschumper and thousands of others like him in North America and Europe are proof that an alternative practice works. It is not only a matter of being chemical-free, it is a practice closer to the natural cycles of plant and animal growth.

The Solution to Ecotoxicity Lies in the Source

What is the possibility that there will be a major switch to the style of farming of Ken Tschumper? One has to be realistic about the economic pressures against that switch. Just as there is a powerful medical – industrial complex with a strong financial stake in selling drugs, equipment and hospitals, there is a parallel agribusiness that has a stake in pesticides, fertilizers and horizon-to-horizon monocropping. Agribusiness supporters take a similar line to that of Aneurin Bevan, who predicted in 1948 that the new medical technology would do away with human disease. They claim that their technology offers the only way to eradicate scarcity and ensure an abundant food supply. They dismiss organic farming as medieval – quaint techniques, poor and uncertain yields.

Yet Tschumper's style of farming depends on something just as exotic technically as genetic engineering; but unlike that spectacular science, it is not done in the laboratory but must be done in the field. As Tschumper says, the farmer must observe closely the signs of nature and fit every aspect of the operation – like the pieces of a jigsaw puzzle into a total picture – into the cycle of crop rotation, composting, manuring, planting and harvesting. No action can be taken without considering how it affects the whole operation. The farmer has to be able to adjust his practices from day to day. These skills are not taught at agricultural colleges, nor are they outlined in official government farm bulletins. Organic farmers have to learn them on their own.

The organic farmers point out that chemical farming requires no such skills, no attention to feedback from nature. Chemical companies provide spray schedules with their products, and the farmer knows that he just has to follow the schedule to control the pest. Automatic spray schedules are like casting a line every day into the same spot in a river in case a trout is swimming past; spray schedules are not sensitive to feedback of whether or not there are any pests there.

Chemical farming exacts a price in environmental contamination, not only of the groundwater, but in residues in food. It is a price that ironically the health-care system is ill-equipped to detect and assess – the studies on contaminants in breast milk are rare. One cannot help being struck by the contrast between the $2 billion a year spent looking for a cure for cancer, and the minuscule amount spent on developing ways of assessing the human health effects of ecotoxicity. This lack of assessment makes it much easier for agribusiness to say there is no evidence of significant health effects from the chemical fallout of that style of farming and to ignore the alternatives to chemical farming.

The American Council on Science and Health, a supporter of agribusiness, announced in a 1989 full-page newspaper advertisement: 'America's food supply is the safest and most plentiful in the world; pesticides deserve much of the credit. If Americans really want to go "back to nature," they will have to coexist with vermin and insects and the diseases they bring. Dismantling the agricultural system will reduce the food supply, forcing consumers to pay the cost.'[15]

It is hard to imagine that when this organization drafted its advertisement, it thought it was contributing to the debate on ecotoxicity. Yet the thinking expressed by such powerful interests profoundly influences the direction of environmental policy. One cannot help but note that the keystone element of this advertisement is the word 'safe', and the implied definition depends on the health-care system's concept of safety. In other words, this special interest group depends heavily on the authority of the health-care system.

Some environmentalists may fret over the biases and influence of such interlocking groups, but we have to realize in a broader sense that, if environmental policy is going to switch to prevention, groups such as the American Council on Science and Health and the health-care system have to be brought into the picture. It is a question of institutional arrangements. The Brundtland Commission complained that governments lacked adequate institutions to solve environmental problems; departments or agencies of the environment by themselves are not effective. Somehow, co-operation among diverse institutions, such as these pressure groups and the health-care system, has to be achieved in the cause of environmental problem solving.

8

Government Attitudes towards Protection of the Environment

The summer of 1988 was not a good year for seals in the North Sea. Almost half of the common harbour seals that live around the coasts of Holland, Germany, Denmark, Norway and Sweden died a fulminating death caused by a virus that normally infects dogs – canine distemper. The disease seemed to be spreading and was infecting populations of seals on Britain's east coast. The fact that a dog virus was killing the animals was news in itself. But what really alarmed marine scientists was the thought that the seals' ability to resist disease was weakened by pollution. Did the seal carcasses washing up on bathing beaches advertise environmental disstress?

The reaction of most government officials to the dead seals was a yawn. An official of the British Ministry of Agriculture, Fisheries and Food assured the public that there are 'no grounds for thinking' that the seal deaths are related to chemical pollutants: 'our people believe it is just one of those things that occurs now and then.'[1]

Environmental problems do not come in neat little packages; they tend to be messy and the indicators of their messiness are not always easy to read. Yet it is these indicators that set in motion the ultimate response. They have to be translated into action. Since all environmental policy and action flow in one way or another from governments, it is the governments' ability or willingness to read the indicators that is going to determine the quality of translation. How does this quality square with the Brundtland Commission's criticism that governments are doing a poor job of environmental protection? Or, to put it another way, that governments have to become more skilful at reading environmental indicators and translating them into action? We examine this

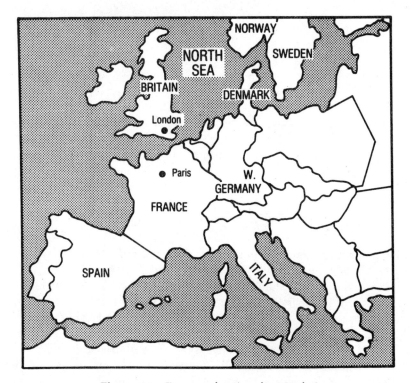

Figure 8.1   Europe, showing the North Sea

question of skill in reading the indicators by looking at some messy environmental problems, starting with the dead seals of the North Sea.

That the North Sea is polluted seems incontestable. Countries surrounding this body of water each year discharge 260,000 tons of liquid industrial waste, 77 million tons of dredged and polluted harbour mud, 5 million tons of sewage sludge, 22,000 tons of lead, 110 tons of mercury and 1,100 tons of cadmium. Another half million tons of nitrogen and phosphate wastes, mainly from agricultural runoff, pours out of the mouth of the Rhine.[2] The total tonnage of waste overwhelms natural cleansing processes, creating a permanently polluted environment for seals and all other North Sea life.

The discharge of pollutants into the North Sea has been going on for centuries, but the sight of seal carcasses littering beaches fanned a smouldering unease that the discharge had become excessive. Bernd Heydemann, Environment Minister for Schleswig-Holstein, the north German state where many of the dead seals washed ashore, was one of the few political leaders to call a polluted sea a polluted sea: 'A principal cause of their deaths is industrial pollution,' he said. 'The immune system of the seals has been injured in a very serious way.'[3] Heydemann's view that the canine virus was able to knock out the seals' weakened immune defences contrasts with the position of the British official that 'it is just one of those things that occurs now and then.' You see the biomedical model operating in the British statement – only proof of a direct connection between pollution and seal deaths would be acceptable. Since 'our people' failed to see a direct connection they could declare with a clear conscience that there was no problem. Heydemann took a more holistic approach – that the disease of the seals was the outcome of many causes and that the way to deal with the problem is do so on a broad front.

Heydemann's willingness to look at a broad pattern of events linking together chemical pollution, immunity, canine virus and seals in the North Sea went beyond the usual government reaction to an environmental issue. He did not agree with the British government's position that there was no problem; to him, the virus-infected seals headlined the more worrisome issue of a deteriorating North Sea ecosystem. The seals were a victim of ecotoxicity.

The public can easily be confused by what appear to be two opposed views of the same environmental picture. It is like two people viewing one of those great panoramic paintings of an eighteenth-century battle with its sweep of columns of soldiers, horses, smoke and cannons. The one viewer takes in the entire sweep, while the other sees only the stirrup of one of the cavalrymen, perhaps unaware that a struggle is taking place at all.

Immunity and Pollution

Well, what is the sweep of the picture that contains dead seals – at least, as seen through the eyes of scientists? That the seals died of canine distemper seems certain. Dr Albert Osterhaus, a veterinary virologist at Holland's National Institute of Public Health and Environmental Protection, said that all the seals tested had antibodies against canine distemper, whereas seals tested in previous years showed no signs of the virus.[4] So apparently exposure to the virus was recent. The disease showed the same symptoms found in infected dogs: watery eyes, thick nasal discharge, inflammation of the lungs, liver and intestines and lesions of the nervous system. Osterhaus, however, was not willing to step beyond his virology and comment on why the seals should all of a sudden be attacked by a virus normally restricted to dogs. However, his colleague in seal research, Ottmar Wassermann, professor of toxicology at the University of Kiel, had no reservation in providing a broader interpretation. He claimed that the large number of chemicals discharged into the North Sea makes traditional cause-and-effect toxicology out of date. He noted the power of many of these chemicals to knock out the immune systems of mice, rabbits and pigs – so why not seals?

Minnie Courtney, a marine biologist at Queen Mary College, London University, said the chemical pollutants actually give a one-two punch to the seals: knock out the immune system and attack the sex organs. She said that high concentrations of PCBs, a common industrial pollutant, were found in the seals' flesh and that the PCBs lower the seals' ability to produce young. It was her view that even if the seals recovered their immunity against the virus, they would be unable to repopulate sufficiently fast to overcome their natural death rate. She believed that only a drastic reduction in dumping of chemical waste into the North Sea would remove the barrier to seal repopulation.[5]

How important are immune defences? Every organism from crab and lobster to seals, dolphins and humans has immune defences against viruses, bacteria and fungi. We all live surrounded by a microscopic world of infectious microbes, but we remain uninfected as long as we remain healthy. This statement sounds circular, but the body's immune defences work only at top efficiency when we are healthy. Tuberculosis was rife among city dwellers of the nineteenth century because their nutrition and living conditions were poor. They fell victim to the tubercular bacillus because their immune system did not defend them. The tubercular bacillus is still with us, but the disease is rare because the stress of poor nutrition and of bad living conditions is all but eliminated.

Efficiency of immune defences for humans and for that matter all organisms falls off as the stress level goes up. Stress for wild animals is often both nutritional and toxic. The kind of pollution that infiltrates the North Sea can change the growth pattern of plants and small animals, the food of larger animals. These animals now find insufficient food or are forced to eat the wrong food, causing nutritional stress. Toxic stress results from the burden of chemical contaminants carried in body tissues. The body tries its best to destroy foreign chemicals, but this is hard work and diverts energy away from important body processes. Moreover, destruction of chemicals takes time, so toxic chemicals reside in the body for hours, days, even years, all the while assaulting delicate biochemical mechanisms needed to support the immune system. The net result:

inadequate nutrition and toxic assault weakens the body's internal strength. Bacteria, fungi and viruses are forever attacking, and eventually one of these microbes breaks through the collapsing immune defences.

Government Insensitivity to a Clogged North Sea

The North Sea seems like a giant toilet bowl that the giant forgot to flush. Eventually the residents around the bowl are going to notice that it is clogged, some residents noticing the problem before others. And even a bowl clogged with chemicals and dead seals may not bother some residents. It depends on how they translate the indicators.

Some take the ecological view and see the human residents as part of the North Sea ecosystem, subject to the same torments as the seals. They see a relationship between seal deaths and the quality of human life. They note that when it comes to maintaining strong immune defences, a human's biology is no different from a seal's and that humans are all caught up in the same ecological web of life. When that web fails to support the life of seals, where does that leave the human population?

Governments, however, say that they have a more pragmatic concept of life. They will say: 'We can't launch expensive cleanup programmes just because seals are dying.' Underlying this position is the assumption that no response is necessary until solid evidence of a connection between pollution and harm knocks one over the head. And that harm has to be directly connected to human health. The British government assured the public that their was no threat to their health from the seals.

There are two issues here, both of which bear on governments' ability to read and translate the indicators. Governments encourage relatively little research into the ecological and health effects of pollution. Some work, of course, is done, as in the case of sick and dying seals, but it is not done on a wide range of species or in a systematic way, and there is practically no study of impacts of the pollution on human health. In other words, governments as yet have not launched programmes that would detail the indicators of environmental stress. As a result, it is easy for government offficials, if they wish, to deny the existence of a problem. A second issue is lack of a mechanism to translate evidence of ecological harm, be it animal or human, into environmental policy decisions. Governments simply have not organized their internal bureaucratic structures to do this.

The situation is equivalent to putting an alleged criminal on trial. The police collect very little evidence of the criminal's deeds, and anyway the judge rejects most of the collected evidence as insignificant. One would consider this to be a strange system of justice; yet governments allow an analogous situation to prevail with respect to the environment.

One reason for this situation can be traced to fragmentation of government bureaucracy. Issues that touch on the environment are spread over many departments and agencies, generally with little co-operation between them. Each sees only a fragment of the whole issue, and fragments in isolation do not look alarming. It is a situation that smothers action. David Suzuki, geneticist and nature broadcaster, says: 'Bureaucratic fragmentation of ecological matters often guarantees that effective action will not take place.'[6]

Let us pursue this theme further in another ecosystem and on another continent: in the Chesapeake Bay on the United States' east coast. We will see how bureaucratic fragmentation of a complex environmental problem in this waterway suppresses understanding of the problem's true dimensions. The indicators are poorly read which leads to weak and sluggish corrective action.

The Chesapeake Ecosystem and the EPA

Chesapeake Bay, like the North Sea, is an identifiable ecosystem, a body of water surrounded by coasts. Once known for its exceptional bounty of fish, the Chesapeake is sliding into the equivalent of a fishless desert, although sports fishermen, ever optimistic, still try to find their favourite fish. The experience of a party of six sports fisherman one summer day in 1988 is typical. The party, guided by Captain Levin Harrison 4th, trolled for striped bass, locally called rockfish. They caught one, a tenpounder, which they threw back because the State levies a fine of $500 and confiscates the boat if the rockfish is kept. The State hopes the species will somehow re-establish itself.

Captain Harrison is the fourth generation of Harrisons to run an inn and boat service on the Chesapeake near Tilghman Island, Maryland. Their inn's dining room was once famous for its mammoth helpings of oysters, perch and rockfish. 'They're all but gone,' said Harrison's father (Levin, the 3rd). 'Traditional fishing in the bay has disappeared. There has been an environmental catastrophe here.'[7] Harrison's assessment seems accurate enough: just twenty-five years ago fishermen caught and ate 2,500 tons of rockfish annually.

Chesapeake oysters have disappeared equally swiftly. In 1977, oystermen landed 6,500 tons; in 1987 they landed 250 tons. A marine parasite has devastated the oyster beds. The parasite, a protozoan known as *Haplosporidium nelsoni*, destroys the oyster's gills and digestive system.

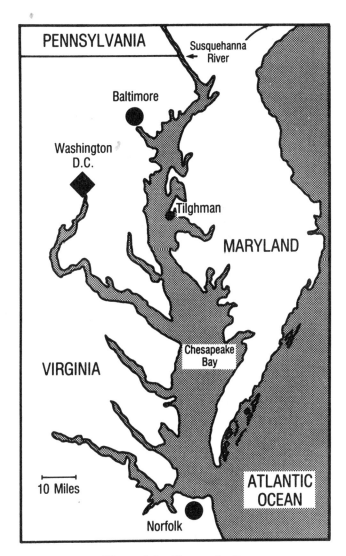

Figure 8.2   Chesapeake Bay

Thomas Faulkner, an oysterman who has 'tonged' for oysters for most of his forty-seven years, said most of the oysters he brings up with his tongs (long scissored poles tipped with baskets) have open shells – dead from the parasite. 'All the bay is good for now is for those damned sailboat people,' he said.[8]

Chesapeake Bay, the United States' largest estuary, extends inland 320 kilometres (195 miles) from the Atlantic, forming a boundary between the states of Virginia and Maryland. Eight major rivers and over 150 creeks empty into the bay, which is ringed with industrial and urban growth, including the cities of Baltimore, Washington DC and Norfolk. These communities have for decades dumped raw sewage, toxic chemicals, waste from livestock feed-farms and fertilizer runoff into the Chesapeake watershed. The EPA in 1983 completed a scientific study that proved what the Harrisons and Faulkner knew all too well: the bay suffers badly from pollution. The study at least galvanized political action, and in 1984 the states of Maryland and Virginia agreed to set up a Chesapeake revitalization plan, co-ordinated by the EPA.

In its role as co-ordinator the EPA analyses the amount of different chemicals in the water at different locations in the estuary. But while their analyses go on year after year, filling up filing cabinets with data, there is no evidence that these data serve as a basis for policy decisions. It has become an embarrassment to the scientists doing the studies. One of them, Christopher D'Elia of the University of Maryland, was quoted as saying that he is happy to receive EPA money to do his research on phosphorus and nitrogen loading of the water, but 'the monitoring can be cut in half and still do the job.' He feels the agency's programme is 'over ambitious and a waste,' because 'it is measuring everything under the sun.'[9]

In fact, since 1983 about all the EPA has done is analyse the bay. A cynic might say that these endless analyses serve to delay hard political decisions that need to be taken if the bay is to be truly cleaned up. The studies give the impression that something is happening, when it is mostly scientists in small boats taking water samples. But before succumbing to cynicism, we should note that such analyses are the underpinnings of environmental agencies and departments in the same way that blood analyses underpin diagnoses by medical doctors.

Environmental agencies do endless analyses because they believe that there are two things they must find out about a polluted water body. First, they believe that only a few of the thousands of pollutants are responsible for death and destruction and these must be identified. It is like being shot at by a machine gun and trying to identify which bullet has your name on it. Secondly, government officials believe that an ecological system, in this case Chesapeake Bay, is capable of digesting a certain amount of pollution. They analyse so they can set threshold levels (standards), the idea being that below a government threshold the pollution is digestible. This is like finding out how much arsenic you can digest without developing violent stomach cramps. In fact you would just as soon not have any arsenic at all.

You see these two beliefs reflected in the statements of environmental officials. Richard Eichbaum, head of Maryland's portion of the Chesapeake Bay Program, was quoted in *Science* magazine as saying that the effects of many of the chemicals dumped into the Bay remain unclear (a favourite phrase of government officials), and without better knowledge it will be difficult to develop effective regulations.[10] What Eichbaum is saying is that we have to know the identity of each chemical and connect a harmful effect, if any, to the chemical. Eichbaum's counterpart in Virginia, Keith Buttleman, was quoted as saying that it is uncertain how clean the Bay must be to restore finfish and shellfish populations.[11] Buttleman clearly believes that the Chesapeake has to be cleaned up only so much and the indicator of cleanliness for him is the return of commercially important fish. The Bay to him is a commercial resource and that is the justification for restoring it. The problem with that attitude is that it leads to cost/benefit analyses where the cost of cleaning up is weighed against the financial benefit of oysters and rockfish.

So the way these government officials read the problem is that a few 'bad actors' among all the chemical pollutants have to be identified and reduced in amount and such action will clean up the estuary. A focus on individual chemicals can lead to gritty, unending argument as happened when d'Elia's research showed that nitrogen stimulates better than phosphorus the growth of great floating mats of algae around the bay.[12] The algae die and sink into the water where they decay, using up all the water's oxygen; fish turn belly up by the thousands of tons. One waterman said, 'blue crabs are so desperate for oxygen they climb onto the pilings of wharves.'

Where is all this nitrogen and phosphorus coming from? Does it matter to the gasping crabs and dead fish which is the greater stimulant of algae? The federal government itself is partly responsible. In the 1970s it gave massive funds to Chesapeake communities to help build sewage treatment plants. The secondary treatment of these plants (primary treatment screens out the lumps) converts human wastes into nitrogen and phosphorus derivatives which pour into Chesapeake Bay, stimulating the growth of algae. State officials at first believed that only phosphorus was responsible for this effect, and they recommended that sewage treatment plants add on phosphorus controls (without removing nitrogen, which requires a more expensive process). No wonder they were dismayed by D'Elia's highly publicized findings that nitrogen, not phosphorus, is the main culprit. The officials saw themselves looking at an additional $2 billion expenditure just to reduce nitrogen discharge.

Why bother upgrading sewage treatment plants? This was the view of Robert Blanco, director of the EPA's Municipal Facilities Division. He pointed out that only about 40 per cent of the nitrogen and phosphorus pollution of the Chesapeake comes from sewage treatment plants, the rest coming from non-point sources. A non-point source is, as the name implies, is a source that does not come out of a discharge pipe. It can be rain, agricultural runoff or the runoff of over-fertilized suburban lawns. 'I don't think it makes a lot of sense to make communities spend a lot of money on these plants,' Blanco was quoted as saying in interview, 'if you're not dealing with 60 percent of the problem.'[13]

Farm Runoff and a Fishless Desert

The major non-point source of Chesapeake pollution is farm runoff into the rivers emptying into Chesapeake Bay.[14] One of the largest is the Susquehanna, which drains half of Pennsylvania's lushly fertilized farmland. You can do something about sewage plants, but how do you control each of 12,000 Pennsylvania farmers who farm the lower Susquehanna and whose runoff represents 41 per cent of the nutrient contribution to Chesapeake Bay? This is the challenge facing Paul Swartz, director of Pennsylvania's Bureau of Soil and Water Conservation. 'Our selling point to the farmer can't be "save the Bay",' said Swartz. 'The bay is not the same to Pennsylvania as it is to Maryland or Virginia.'[15]

Part of Swartz's job is to persuade farmers to practise conservation and use just enough fertilizer to prevent an excess that then becomes runoff. But the State has given him a small office of four people and no power. The farmers can literally kick Swartz off their farms. Far removed from talk of rockfish, oysters and algal blooms, they are more interested in crop yield, which, in their view, demands lavish application of nitrogen and phosphorus fertilizer.

Runoff is more than excessive fertilization; it includes the waste of farm animals. The American farm animal population produces five times the body waste of the country's human population,[16] and as far as the environment is concerned, urine is urine, faeces is faeces, regardless of its source. The storybook picture of mixed farms where the farmer recycles the manure by spreading it on the fields all but disappeared after the Second World War. Most crops are grown on farms without animals. The animals, on the other hand, are compacted in feedlots or barns, their feed trucked from distant states. (Maryland has one of the largest concentrations of chickens in the United States.) There are no crops to absorb the wastes, and the nitrogen and phosphorus from these wastes cascades into streams and groundwater. It is small wonder that Robert Blanco pleaded for a perspective on the whole waste problem and for not believing that upgrading sewage treatment plants for human wastes will prevent the deterioration of Chesapeake Bay.

You see in this situation an example of a major defect in government environmental policy: the many cracks through which issues fall into oblivion. Governments have not only failed to create environmental departments with teeth, they have failed to develop and co-ordinate an overall environmental policy. Blanco, the EPA chief, can only issue press releases; his hands are tied. As an EPA official he cannot tell farmers to use less fertilizer, and, in any event, just telling farmers to use less fertilizer without giving them an incentive to adjust their whole farming technique is futile. You cannot tell a chemical-intensive farmer to give up his large fertilizer input (with the risk of a drop in yield) any more than you can easily persuade him to give up pesticides. Could Blanco and other EPA officials then tell their bureaucratic counterparts in the Department of Agriculture to force farmers to stop the runoff? Hardly: the weak position of the EPA in the United States federal government gives it little influence over other agencies.

The problem is that agriculture, like other government sectors concerned with production, puts environment at the bottom of its priorities. Agriculture, prompted by agribusiness, views its role as producing two blades of grass where one grew before and wraps itself in policy questions of subsidies and yields. Questions of agriculture runoff and pesticide residues are entertained only as long as they do not get in the way of production. Swartz's official mission in the farmlands of Pennsylvania was actually soil conservation, and his personal interest in runoff was incidental to that mission.

Should Ecosystems be Immortal?

Ecosystems have a living quality, inasmuch as the whole ecosystem can be thought of as a single organism, and, like such an organism, can be killed by excessive stress. But death comes slowly to an ecosystem and early indicators of stress are difficult for governments to read. The indicators, however, become more blatant the closer to death the system comes. We could, in fact, construct a fanciful index – the sitting-on-a-tack index. In the early stages of ecosystem stress, the indicators are subtle, the tack barely starting to penetrate. But as stress becomes excessive, the tack penetrates more and more. How far does this environmental tack have to penetrate into the hides of politicians and bureaucrats before they say 'ouch' and start to respond? We have no answer to that question because we are experiencing for the first time in modern history the overstress of the global ecosystem. Governments as yet have not really developed the means to respond to early stage indicators; in fact, they also respond poorly to later stage indicators, almost as if they were waiting until the end appears imminent before making an attempt to reverse the deterioration. Ironically, the cost of effective counteraction skyrockets, the longer governments wait to say 'ouch'.

This attitude of waiting almost until the bell tolls has its parallel in the health-care system, although reluctance to throw in money is not evident. With about one third of the US national health-care budget spent during the last year of everyone's life, critics say that much of the expensive medical care lavished on the aged could be avoided by better targeted spending, particularly on preventive measures, at the other end of the age spectrum.

Although there is a parallel between the biology of a ecosystem and that of a single human, ecosystems are not supposed to die; they are immortal, at least on the timescale of human history. Yet the attitude of waiting for advanced deterioration and then deciding whether or not to apply cure extends from human medicine to issues of the environment. It is this waiting that exasperates many environmentalists. They read environmental indicators more clearly; they have thin skins, are less tolerant to the pain of the penetrating environmental tack than government bureaucrats and politicians. Much of the argument between environmentalists and governments, in fact, is over how much the environmental tack has to inch in before action is triggered.

Solid Garbage

Part of the difficulty of dealing with environmental issues lies in defining the problem. It is usually defined as some end result, such as dead seals, explosive growth of algae or lack of oysters. There is a general failure to define the problem with all its deep connections, something that is necessary if preventive action is to be mounted. The spoiling of the North Sea and Chesapeake ecosystems is due to the waste of industries and people. If that is the case, then all we need to do is stop dumping the wastes. But this is not simple. First we have to define wastes, and that definition may not be so easy as it seems at first glance. Let us start with household garbage.

Most US cities have an agency that accepts used clothing, furniture, toys and other home discards, which handicapped workers clean and repair for resale. But the discards in some cities, particularly where householders pay for garbage collection, have taken on an air of grottiness. Carl Sieben is the head sorter in one such agency, Goodwill Industries, Harrison, NJ, which has eighty collection boxes throughout several neighbouring New Jersey cities. His job is to sort the collected articles into streams for the plant's workers. He said recent collections included a suitcase of mayonnaise, empty vodka bottles, half a rotting deer, 'tons' of soft drink cans, and matted wads of disposed nappies, some of the 16 billion disposable nappies carrying 2.8 million tons of baby faeces and urine that wind up in US garbage each year.[17] In fact, 40 per cent of Goodwill's collections is now household garbage, compared to 5 per cent five years ago. It has become so expensive to have your trash hauled away, said Sieben (a householder in Plainfield, NJ pays $38 monthly) that it is no wonder people routinely use Goodwill collection boxes as a free dump.

Garbage collection and disposal are traditionally handled by local authorities. But the sheer volume of garbage cities produce is rapidly exceeding the authorities' ability to deal with it, and clandestine dumping in charity collection boxes is but a symptom of the problem. Modern cities generate 0.7 to 1.0 ton of solid waste each year for each resident. (This figure does not include industrial waste, which amounts to another ton per year per citizen.) And the volume swells as cities grow, and people individually generate more waste. The waste is far from benign and no matter how it is disposed of – buried in a landfill, dumped at sea or incinerated – it exacts a painful cost from the environment. But environmental agencies of central governments have adopted a hands-off attitude towards city garbage. City managers, struggling to dispose of their day-to-day collections, receive little guidance and certainly no overall environmental strategy from these agencies. Like sheets of paper in a wind storm, these city managers find themselves helpless to cope with issues they did not create. There are three aspects to the problem: the costs of garbage collection and disposal, like health-care costs, are climbing far more rapidly than the rate of inflation (costs in the United States doubled in the three-year period, 1984–7); locally available space for landfill is all but gone; and all forms of disposal – dumping, incineration – are perceived as hazardous to human health.

Cities sometimes reach for desperate solutions. Trash-rich cities on the American east coast, for example, tried to make a deal to bury 1.25

million tons a year of their trash in the apparently trash-poor English counties of Cornwall and Cheshire. These two counties already have a thriving business burying garbage from Holland, Australia and other countries at a cost of about $16 a ton, compared with as much as $100 a ton for disposal in the United States. The Manchester Ship Canal Company, a partner in the plan to bury American garbage, responding to objections from local residents, said that trash is trash and the disposal meets government standards.[18] Whether or not this deal is consummated, the British Isles seem an unlikely place to bury American garbage.

The British will say that America, with its enormous land mass, has plenty of room to bury its garbage, but although cities look longingly at the seemingly vacant rural areas, residents of most communities with available land, like the English citizens, say: 'Not In My Backyard'. They will do everything they can to prevent foreign garbage from coming into their community for burial. The attitude of most communities has become: 'if you produce it, get rid of it within your own boundaries.' Such objections are a headache for big cities with a small amount of vacant land suitable for a landfill. American cities bury 80 per cent of their household garbage, but the EPA says that half of America's cities will run out of landfill space before 2000.[19]

So, with inter-community transport of garbage blocked, cities are turning to incineration, whereby the whole garbage mix is dumped into an incinerator and burnt. But 30–60 per cent of the original weight is left as ash, so all the city has done is reduce the amount of its solid waste by about half. Moreover, the EPA predicts that Americans will double their production of household garbage by 2000, so even if it is all incinerated, by then the amount of ash will equal what is being buried today. Moreover, both the ash and the stack emissions from an incinerator are hazardous. The incinerator is just a big furnace, but its fuel mix is as diverse as household and industrial wastes, and highly toxic substances are produced in the violent chemistry of combustion. Old credit cards, floor tiles, plastic raincoats and records made of polyvinyl chloride, react with food residues to produce dioxins, among the most toxic substances known.

Local solutions are just not working. The volume of garbage creeps ever upwards while city officials and citizens argue over the respective merits of incineration, landfills, burial at sea or recycling. Recycling! That seems like a good solution. Recycling, however, just increases the number of times an item or substance is used; it does not get rid of the substance. And recycling is unable to handle all the garbage. Machida City, Japan, has one of the most intensive and innovative recycling programmes in the world, yet has only been able to cut the city's solid waste by half.[20]

The solution lies in the questions: Why do we produce waste? Could we live a modern lifestyle without producing waste? These questions are better raised by central governments, but to do so questions the fundamental way we conduct our lives.

The Disposable Razor Lasts Four Centuries

Consider the plastic razor. The disposable plastic razor symbolizes the problem of trying to cure rather than prevent. In 1988 Americans discarded two billion plastic razors, part of the plastic waste that accounts for 25 per cent of the volume of solid waste. Each razor, used for one minute, lasts for four centuries.

A sailboater travelling the length of the American east coast, 100 miles offshore, reported that he was never out of sight of plastic debris. Marine biologists estimate that every year two million sea birds and 100,000 sea lions, porpoises, whales and other sea mammals strangle or choke on the 639,000 plastic bags and containers tossed into the oceans every day. Countless fish drown in an estimated 150,000 tons of plastic fishing line set adrift every year. The image of this innocent slaughter at sea prompts demands that plastic be made biodegradable, especially plastics used in packaging materials. Technically, plastics can be made that degrade in sunlight or are attacked by common soil bacteria. But plastic compacted in a dump is not exposed to sunlight, and inside the dump there is relatively little of the moisture or oxygen which bacteria need to carry out their work. So biodegradability is not a simple answer. Also, biodegradability works at cross-purposes with recycling.

Plastics come in a large variety of synthetic types, all jumbled together in garbage. The Heinz plastic ketchup bottle alone contains five different plastics. Nevertheless, engineers are finding ways to recycle plastic mixtures, what they call dirty plastic, into products like plastic beams, park benches, boat docks and roofing material. It is becoming a profitable business because the raw material – the waste plastic – costs about half as much as new plastic. The recycling engineers, however, are horrified by the thought that biodegradable plastics will start finding their way into the garbage stream, because it is difficult to separate the different plastics and their final products are exposed to sunlight and moisture. Who wants a park bench or a dock that biodegrades?

It is hard to imagine life without plastic. There is hardly anything you use that does not contain some form of plastic. The major problem in dealing with plastics is absence of a comprehensive policy with respect to use and the types of plastics made. Environmental agencies have failed to develop an overview of the entire plastics industry that charts the manufacture, use and ultimate disposal of each item. In other words, when a new plastic item is to be manufactured the question needs to be asked: How will the item be used and, most importantly, where will it end up? If ultimate disposal is a problem then the item should not be made. Such an overview is not now taken and plastics manufacturers are able to manufacture anything they wish, taking no responsibility for the fact that it may wind up wrapped around a dolphin, stuck in a pelican's gullet or sitting in a garbage mound four centuries from now.

Cradle to Grave

Cradle-to-grave control: this is what some environmentalists call the concept of controlling products from manufacture to disposal, and it applies not only to plastic but to everything we produce. This is not a definition of waste that city managers can be expected to put into practice. It is a concept so sweeping that only central governments would have the power and resources to make a plan of this nature work.

The cradle-to-grave concept, stripped of production and waste figures, is something schoolchildren learn about in their science classes, but politicians seem to forget. It is the simple but fundamental law of nature: the conservation of mass. We are unable to destroy anything; we can only change its form. This lesson was burned into Brendan Sexton, New York City's Sanitation Commissioner, as he gazed at a pyramid of city trash ten times larger than the great pyramid of Cheops. 'Fresh Kills [the name of the dump], he said, 'is the living, working proof that we throw away as much as we consume.'[21] Take this logic further: everything we produce in our society eventually becomes waste of some form. That is, everything we produce is eventually discarded. This is a true definition of waste.

If you want to get some concept of the growing problem of waste disposal, look at the production figures. The United States produced 27.1 million tons of all types of plastics in 1987, which some day will be 27.1 million tons of plastic garbage. That is 100 kg of plastic garbage for each inhabitant. And that figure will double by the time today's baby in its disposable nappy reaches college age. Our industrial societies are committed to a relentless rise in production. The industrial world produces seven times more goods today than it did in 1950, and there is reason to believe that world production will expand at about the same rate: doubling every thirteen years. The space for waste disposal, however – the oceans, the air, the land – remains the same. So we are literally becoming engorged on our own production.

The disposable nappy symbolizes the dilemma. Introduced about 1970, it has become the indispensable friend of young parents. But environmentalists view it differently. 'It's a perfect case where we're using a disposable product that costs more than a re-usable product, is more environmentally dangerous and uses up nonrenewable resources,' said Jeanne Wirka, a policy analyst with the Environmental Action Foundation, Washington, DC.[22] She believes that either the companies should make biodegradable nappies or the government should promote use of cotton nappies.

A baby is changed 6–10 thousand times before it is toilet trained, producing some two tons of soiled disposable nappies. That tonnage could be replaced by a small stack of cotton nappies. If modern parents dislike rewashing nappies they could subscribe to a nappy service that provides a clean nappy for about 15 cents, as opposed to the price of 22 cents for a disposable one. Most nappy services, however, have been driven out of business by the surge to disposables.

You do not hear politicians discussing the merits of disposable versus cotton nappies: that is part of the environmental dilemma. Disposable nappies have grown into a $3.3 billion-a-year business in the United States without government officials ever pondering the meaning of the word 'disposable'. There is no attempt to see the problem from the cradle to the grave. Disposable nappy manufacturers argue that their products occupy only 2 per cent of the space on garbage trucks and that therefore, nappies make up only a small part of the total problem of solid waste. It seems an irresistible argument; but then, plastic razor manufacturers can argue that their product occupies only a small part of the dump, so can the ketchup bottle makers, the battery makers and so on. Governments simply are not organized to think in comprehensive terms.

Fractured government authority along traditional lines of water planning, industrial development, social planning, waste disposal, etc., to say nothing of divisions between a central government and State and city governments, does not work well when it comes to addressing problems of ecosystem degradation. Now, this is not a plea for some kind of ecosystem tsar. Cities can remain in charge of their garbage, but what is needed is comprehensive cradle-to-grave planning that, in effect, brings together manufacturers and garbage commissioners. This is where we need some vision from central governments. But one is driven to the conclusion that governments have inadequate internal arrangements and weak policy-making mechanisms for reading the indicators of environmental stress and for co-ordinating systematic and comprehensive planning. They just do not have the nerve endings to feel the penetrating environmental tack. It is fair to say that without elevation of environmental issues to a top position in government priorities and a willingness to look at the cradle-to-grave realities of production, North Sea seals, Chesapeake oysters and cotton nappies have a limited future.

9

Acid Rain, Ozone and the Resiliency Principle

'Decay is not a steady, continuous loss of material: for many years, there may be little visible cracking or erosion. The rock then reaches a critical threshold and fails. One extreme event, such as a long frost, may prompt premature failure from fatigue.'[1] This decay, described by Bernard Smith and Brian Whalley, geochemists at Queens University, Belfast, and Vasco Fassina, chief chemist at the Laboratorio Scientifico della Misericordia, Venice, is crumbling the cathedrals, palaces, public buildings and bridges of Europe. Workers sweep up 52 tons of masonry dust from around Cologne Cathedral every year. The whole city of Venice, once a variegated spectacle of marble and Istrian limestone, has passed the critical threshold mentioned by these scientists. Once that happens, they say, 'deterioration is often rapid.'

Their description of the stonework of a building that looks so solid yet is decaying from within could be the description of a deteriorating biology. The man in his fifties, robust on the outside but arteries decaying on the inside, unable to resist some extreme event like a blood clot, is felled by a heart attack. The heart attack could have been prevented by paying attention earlier to lifestyle. The point these scientists wished to get across applies equally to the living: it is easy to clean a scaly cathedral or undergo heart bypass surgery, but the remaining rock is already decaying and the 'new' arteries soon build up their scaly plaques. The decay in both instances can only be arrested by dealing with the causes.

If we wanted to summarize these observations in the form of a principle, we could call it the resiliency principle. Natural systems, be they the stone facing of a cathedral, a heart muscle or an estuary like the Chesapeake, have a built-in resilience to stress, which initially can be accommodated without any apparent change in the system; but unceasing stress grinds down resilience, imperceptibly at first, but gradually accelerating. By the time the system is noticeably deteriorating, the reservoir of resilience may be used up.

As we found in the previous chapter, the political processes of our governments are poorly organized to respond to early signs of decay; and usually, for that matter, to later and more striking signs too. There is always argument over what the signs mean, and regardless of what may be said, two questions permeate the argument. Is, or is not, the system resilient enough to accommodate continuing stress? How far can the system be driven before the situation becomes irretrievable? The difficulty governments have in addressing these two questions is evident in two world-size environmental issues: acid rain and erosion of the ozone shield.

Acid rain (also called acid deposition) is a cause of crumbling stone buildings, decaying forests and sterile lakes. It is a complex situation that confounds governments' desire to establish direct cause-and-effect linkages – one excuse for inaction. In the case of an eroding ozone shield, however, a direct linkage is recognized – chlorofluorocarbons (CFCs) cause the erosion. But even here one finds hesitancy and timidity. In both cases, policy-makers have difficulty in understanding the principle: there is only so much resiliency in nature's bank.

Acid Rain

'The acid rain problem in Canada and the United States is small and does not require urgent action,' said John Herrington, Secretary of Energy in the Reagan administration. 'The known problem is small; I think we're handling it well,' he told a congressional committee in 1986.[2]

How small a problem is it? For an answer, let us start in a remote camp near the village of Vermillion Bay in north-western Ontario. This isolated and unpretentious collection of trailers, cabins and laboratories is the site of one of the world's most innovative centres for study of the effects of acid rain on global ecosystems. Every summer, some fifty scientists and their families live here. The director, David Schindler of Canada's Department of Fisheries and Oceans, says the region is ideal for controlled studies of the effects of acid rain because it is remote, uncluttered by habitation or tourists, and there are dozens of small lakes with similar ecosystems.

Schindler's studies started in 1976 with one of the lakes, simply designated Lake 223. The plan was to acidify the lake slowly and see what happened. Scientists added a measured amount of sulphuric acid, dumping it from a small boat and letting it disperse in the wash of the propeller. These particular lakes have a small amount of buffering capacity that neutralizes the acid, and in the first summer, the acidity of the water didn't change. Schindler's team repeated the acid loading the following summer, and as buffering capacity was limited, Lake 223 became mildly acidic.

Scientists measure acidity on the pH scale, where 7 is neutral and the acidity becomes greater as the number becomes smaller. The pH scale is logarithmic: acidity goes up by a factor of ten for a decrease of each pH unit; that is, pH 6 is ten times more acidic than pH 7. The normal pH of Lake 223 was 6.8; by the second summer it had dropped to 6.1, which seems like a small change but in fact, represents a five-fold increase in acidity. All organisms are able to resist changes in the acidity of their environment by means of internal buffering mechanisms, but this buffering varies: some organisms are more resilient than others. The increase in acidity in the second summer caused noticeable shifts in the algae populations of Lake 223. The normal brown algae began to disappear and acid-resistant green algae began to appear.

The next summer, when Schindler and his team increased the acidity to pH 5.8, they saw major effects on fish. Fishes' reproductive organs are highly sensitive to the stress of pollution. Trout embryos began to die, and the fathead minnow, a food for larger fish, failed to reproduce. Some species of crustaceans began to disappear.

In the summer of 1979, the fourth year of the experiment, the acidity was increased to pH 5.6 (only three times more acidic than the previous summer). The fathead minnow all but disappeared, the white sucker began to disappear, and the opossum shrimp, a major food source for lake trout, vanished. The shells of crayfish, a shrimp-like bottom crawler, softened. The green algae now grew in squishy mats along the shoreline of what was once a clear lake.

The following summer, Schindler's team added more sulphuric acid; the acidity increased to a pH of 5.4. More species of crustaceans vanished and the lake trout failed to lay hatchable eggs. Pearl dace, a small minnow, appeared in large numbers. These fish are more resistant to acid, and without competition from the fathead minnow, they throve. The crayfish with their weakened shells were infested with parasites.

In 1981 the researchers increased the acidity of Lake 223 to 5.1 (fifty times the original acidity of pH 6.8). The white sucker and crayfish failed to reproduce. Leeches and mayflies vanished and the few remaining adult trout, their fins sloughed off, looked like eels. The bottom of the lake was covered with masses of gelatinous, beach-ball size clumps of green algae.[3] The population of pearl dace, the last of the fish to survive, began to decline. The biological resiliency of this lake ecosystem was exhausted. There was no strength left to resist any more incursion of acid.

Schindler's reason for slowly acidifying Lake 223 was to demonstrate that even in the early stages of acid rain fallout the biology of a lake suffers. Many critics, sceptical of the effects of acid rain, say they catch fish in a lake so what's the problem? But Schindler, in studying the total ecological web of the lake, sees the gradual destruction of that web. It is like shooting holes in a spider's web; eventually the web fails and can no longer support the spider.

Schindler also keeps track of the effects of acid rain on the lakes of North America. He has found 100,000 lakes in eastern Canada and 6,531 lakes in the north-eastern United States suffering 'biological depletion' – Schindler's way of describing early signs of ecological decay; the normal food chain is upset. 'Even though some of the organisms aren't aesthetically very beautiful, there is reason for concern,' he said in interview. 'For instance, you might be happy to see the leeches disappear, but that affects the food chain.'[4]

The natural resiliency of the North American ecology is being used up. How far does deterioration have to go before effective steps are taken to turn the situation around? The answer is more political than scientific.

Sulphur Dioxide and the Political Acid Rain Axis

First, where is all the acid coming from? A lot of it originated millions of years ago. All living organisms contain sulphur, and when the convulsions of our distant geological past compressed the earth's vegetation into fossil fuel, the sulphur remained. As a result, coal and petroleum contain 1–5 per cent by weight sulphur, which when the fuel burns becomes sulphur dioxide, a pungent, toxic gas. Most commercial boilers lack scrubbers to remove the sulphur dioxide, and it blows straight up the smokestack, where it undergoes an atmospheric reaction. It dissolves in raindrops forming a dilute solution of sulphuric acid, the same acid that Schindler dumped into Lake 223.

Sulphur dioxide represents only about half the source of acid rain; other major sources are automobile exhausts, stationary furnaces and forest fires which generate nitrogen oxides (NOx). I focus here on sulphur dioxide to illustrate the political and mental roadblocks to dealing with acid rain.

The political axis of the acid rain issue in North America extends along a west–east line between Cheshire, Ohio and a cloud research station on top of Whiteface Mountain in New York State, a distance of 920 km (570 miles). Cheshire is the site of two huge coal-fired electric power plants, the Kyger Creek and the James M. Gavin. Together, they discharge about 570,000 metric tons (625,000 tons) of sulphur dioxide annually, the single largest emission in the United States. These plants and dozens of others are located on the Ohio River as it winds through the mid-western states of West Virginia, Ohio, Kentucky, Indiana and Illinois. It is the sulphur dioxide epicentre of the United States. The sulphur dioxide from all these plants, thrown high in the air by thousand-foot smokestacks, blows in an easterly direction into Canada, New England and New York State – including the 1,600 m (4,867 ft) high Whiteface cloud research station.

The mid-western electric utility companies claim that their pollution does not carry that far and that acid precipitation in the north-east comes from local sources. But Liaquat Husain, a chemist working at the Whiteface cloud research station said that he could 'fingerprint' each source of sulphur dioxide and show clearly that 70 per cent of all sulphur dioxide blowing past the station was from the mid-western sulphur dioxide epicentre.[5]

The electric power plants cluster in the Ohio river valley because they feed nearby industry and because they are close to major coalfields in West Virginia and Kentucky, where the coal mined has a high sulphur content. The coal and electric utility companies, supported by politicians from these areas, present a formidable lobby that has successfully blocked any laws to force the coal-fired plants to emit less sulphur dioxide. The issue in their view is cost, not technology: scrubbers can be installed in the plants that spray a neutralizing solution of dissolved lime into the stack gases, removing some 90–95 per cent of the sulphur dioxide. The pollution, however, is in this case transferred to the ground as a lime–sulphur sludge. The amount is prodigious: all the coal-fired electric power stations of the United States, if equipped with scrubbers, would produce each year enough sludge to cover the city of Washington DC to a depth of 3 m (10ft). In fifty years the sludge would reach the top of the Washington monument. Nevertheless, in terms of overall pollution, it is easier to deal with sulphur on the ground than in the air. The US government believes this, and President Bush in the summer of 1989 introduced proposals that would force the electric utilities to start scrub-bing. The coal–electric lobby was not pleased. The American Electric

Power Company, which serves seven states, responded that this acid rain proposal would wreck the economy. It would make the building of new plants impossible and would bar existing plants from running at full power, according to W. S. White, president of the company.[6] But the EPA disputed White's doomsday scenario, saying that the technology for pollution control is available and cost-effective.

So there the matter stands: much argument, while the lakes of North America become increasingly, in Schindler's words, biologically impoverished.

The Environmental Fallout of Acid Rain

Acid rain is a worldwide problem, and the damage is accelerating. Ancient Mayan temples in the Yucatan peninsula are eroding at an accelerating rate; the destruction in the past ten years has been particularly savage, according to Richard Adams, an archeologist studying the sites.[7] The rain forests of Central America and Africa are being damaged by acid rain. Forest damage in Europe has been reported for several decades: *Waldsterben* – forest death – is what they call it in West Germany, where a government forest survey in 1982 found 8 per cent of trees were damaged by acid rain. One year later, the survey showed a damage rate of 34 per cent in the heavily forested regions of Bavaria and Baden-Württemburg. Half of the acid rain comes from outside West German borders, some of it from France and Britain; but these two countries, like the upwind states of the United States, are resisting doing anything about their emissions.

This resistance stems from at least three factors. First, the distance between emitters and the recipients of the acid rain can be large, often crossing national boundaries, and it is easy to ignore the complaints of neighbours; secondly, it is impossible to draw a direct link between a particular smokestack and a particular lake or tree; and thirdly, there is minimal information about direct effects on human health traceable to acid rain; the assumption being that humans are much more resilient than fathead minnows or spruce trees. All three factors can be summed up as a refusal to take an ecological, or preventive, approach to the problem, a failure to acknowledge how a living system, whether a lake or a tree or a human, responds to relentless stress.

Consider what one forester, Glen Likens, has to say about such stress on forests: 'When you're tired, you're more likely to catch a cold, and trees are the same way.' he said. Likens, director of the Institute of Ecosystem Studies, Millbrook, NY, was speaking of a forest his group had been studying for the past twenty-five years in the White Mountains of New Hampshire (the downwind end of the American acid rain axis). The tiredness of the trees, according to Likens, is caused by multiple stresses including various forms of air pollution. The trees could probably handle one or two forms of stress, but too many and they succumb to some disease they would otherwise resist. 'It's not just acid rain,' Likens added. 'It's ozone and lead in rainfall and droughts and defoliating insects like gypsy moths.'[8]

Contrast Likens's thinking with that of Richard Lugar, a United States Senator from Indiana, an upwind state with several coal-fired power plants: 'The effects of acid rain are uncertain.' In Lugar's view, if scientists cannot say precisely what the sources of acid rain are and what the connection between the source and damage is, then they should not 'lay the burden for reduction of emissions of sulfur and nitrogen oxides on the utilities of the Midwest.'[9] Lugar looks for the direct connection and is saying: without evidence of the connection, do nothing. Likens points out that when a living organism such as a tree is subjected to acid rain or other stress it becomes weakened and unable to defend itself from insect pests or disease. The trees, subjected to multiple stresses, succumb; there is no one cause of the death. Certainly, if the coal-fired utilities install acid scrubbers this will not remove all the stresses; but at least it will remove one of the contributing causes.

Lugar's neighbour from Tennessee, Senator Albert Gore Jr, has no trouble in understanding the import of Likens's observation. Gore supports strongly the Brundtland Commission's belief that if governments are ever going to switch environmental policy to prevention they will have to get off the one-cause/one-effect track and stop waiting for scientists to unravel all the linkages. We haven't time, he says: 'The [environmental] crisis is so different from anything before that it is hard to believe it is real. We seize scientific uncertainties, however small, as excuses for inaction.'[10] Gore's plea frames nature's resiliency principle: you cannot wait until the last stages of decay and then expect recovery.

The Ozone Shield

Donald Hodel, Interior Secretary in the Reagan administration, suggested that the way to deal with the more intense ultraviolet light reaching earth because of an eroding ozone shield was to apply stronger sunscreen lotions and wear protective clothing. He said this on learning of the predicted increase in skin cancer from increased exposure to the ultraviolet light. His suggestion brought a scathing rejoinder from

Michael Oppenheimer and Daniel Dudek of the Environmental Defense Fund: '[It is] akin to issuing gas masks to mitigate air pollution.'[11]

While most environmental issues are multi-causal and full of uncertainty, here is one offering a single cause of a single effect that is reasonably certain. The effect, human cancer, is not contested and the cause, the industrial chemicals, CFCs, is also not contested. As in the case of acid rain, a major industry is affected by a solution to ozone erosion. But because a direct human health effect is the outcome, the driving force for corrective action is sufficient to secure industry co-operation.

The political issue in this case is time; there is no understanding that each minute the ozone shield continues to erode, the risk of irreversible failure of the shield increases. William Reilly, head of the EPA, noted further that we lack good policy-making structures to respond rapidly enough.[12] The political process takes too long: 'the earth could be destabilized fairly rapidly,' he said, 'in ways we do not yet have the legal or institutional means to address.'[13]

Enough of politics for the moment; now some science. What is so important about the ozone shield? First, a few facts. The lower atmosphere, the part we experience as wind, clouds and rain, extends to the maximum height commercial jets fly, 12 km (7.2 miles). Above this layer lies the rarefied air of the stratosphere, which contains ozone, an augmented form of oxygen whose molecules each consist of three atoms of oxygen compared to the normal two. The ozone envelops the world like an eggshell, extending in a layer 12 to 40 km (7.2–24 miles) above the earth's surface. This 30 km (18 mile) layer, however, is so dilute that, if it were compressed to the pressure of air at sea level, it would be the thickness of window glass.

The ozone layer, like window glass, transmits visible light, and, again like window glass, it blocks ultraviolet light. Ultraviolet light is hazardous to all living organisms because it damages the cell's genetic material, the DNA. The damage can be lethal: skin cancer in humans and large-scale destruction of plant life. A small amount of ultraviolet light actually reaches the earth's surface, but organisms have adapted to this. Light-skinned people develop tans, and if there is genetic damage in skin cells, biochemical mechanisms repair the damage. Plants also have defensive mechanisms against a low level of ultraviolet light. But as the ozone layer becomes thinner, the amount of ultraviolet light transmitted soars, and neither humans nor plants can adapt rapidly enough to the increased amounts.

It is estimated that the extra ultraviolet radiation from a 5 per cent decrease in the ozone layer will increase the incidence of human skin cancer by 25 per cent. The yield of soybeans, a major world food crop, will drop by 25 per cent.[14] Other plants, such as the photosynthetic plankton, will suffer. Damage to these plankton would knock out the foundation of the ocean food chain because they are eaten by small fish, molluscs and krill which in turn are food for large fish, whales and penguins. Donat Haber, a marine biologist in West Germany, has said: 'When you expose a population of these organisms [plankton] to ultra-violet light, they die within a few hours.'[15]

The ozone layer has long interested atmospheric scientists, and it was a British team working at Halley Bay in the Antarctic which noticed in 1982 a strange erosion of the ozone above the Antarctic. Erosion continued and by 1985 the disappearance of ozone was so great that the scientists began to talk about a hole in the ozone layer the size of Antarctica: if a hard-boiled egg represents the earth, and the shell the ozone layer, and you peel off a portion of the shell at one end the size of your thumbnail, that gap is equivalent to the ozone hole.

The British scientists noticed something else; the amounts of CFCs in the stratosphere of the Antarctic underwent a steady increase matching the decline of the ozone. It was not by accident they measured the amount of CFCs, because in the early 1970s Sherwood Rowland and Mario Molina of the University of California at Irvine had proposed that the man-made CFCs penetrate the stratosphere and cause destruction of ozone. The chemical companies that make CFCs ridiculed the Rowland–Molina proposal: 'Where is your evidence?' they said. But now, some ten years later, the British scientists came up with evidence that Rowland and Molina are right, that the CFCs do cause destruction of ozone.[16]

CFCs were invented sixty years ago by a Dupont Chemical Company scientist, Thomas Midgley, who had been told by his bosses to find a safe substitute for ammonia, then used as a refrigerant gas. Ammonia is highly toxic, and leaking refrigerators caused many deaths. Midgley's CFCs (the Dupont trademark is Freon) are relatively non-toxic and non-flammable, and have been used for refrigeration ever since. Later, with the invention of the aerosol spray can, CFCs became the commonly used propellant, and by the 1970s about three quarters of CFC production was used to propel foamy shaving cream, underarm deodorant and spray paints. This so-called trivial use was banned in 1978 in the United States, Canada, Sweden and Norway, but not in the rest of Europe.

The problem is that after use the CFCs escape and enter the atmosphere. The world's yearly production of some 700,000 metric tons (770,000 tons) becomes another 700,000 metric tons added to the atmosphere. It takes only about two years from production until the CFC is used and vented to the atmosphere. But unlike sulphur dioxide and nitrogen oxides, CFCs are insoluble in water and do not wash out of the lower atmosphere; instead, they wend slowly upwards and in five to ten years reach the stratosphere and the ozone layer, where they can persist for several human lifetimes. The CFCs in one can of foamy shaving cream will over the next 100 years or so destroy twenty tons of ozone.

If any doubt remained among scientists as to what the CFCs were doing to the Antarctic ozone, they were dispelled in the late winters of 1986 and 1987. Alerted by the British discovery of the ozone hole, scientists of several nations converged on the Antarctic. The main base of operations was the South American city of Punta Arenas, located at the southern tip of Chile. Two NASA (United States National Aeronautics and Space Administration) aircraft flying from Punta Arenas made several flights over the Antarctic from mid-August to the end of September each year. One aircraft, a converted U-2 spy plane, called an ER-2, flew at the upper limit at which a jet can fly, 20 km (12 miles), automatically collecting air, which was analysed by on-board instruments for ozone and CFC content. The second aircraft, a converted DC-8 jetliner, flew at an altitude of 12 km (7 miles) carrying a crew of forty scientists and a more complex set of instruments than the ER-2. The many flights of the two aircraft in the two years, together with information from satellite and ground stations, provided enough proof that the ozone hole is man-made and that CFCs are the culprits.[17]

The Antarctic ozone hole was just the start. Following the 1986 and 1987 Antarctic expeditions, in spring 1988 the world's atmospheric scientists converged on Snowmass, Colorado, to compare their data for the entire ozone layer. They concluded that erosion is not confined to the Antarctic ozone hole: the ozone layer worldwide has shrunk by 2.5 per cent in the last decade.[18]

It is not the CFCs themselves that destroy the ozone: they slowly break down in the stratosphere, releasing chlorine, and this chemical does the dirty work. The CFCs, in effect, act as a long-term reservoir for the chlorine, which acts as a catalyst: that is, a trace of chlorine causes destruction of a large amount of ozone.[19]

CFCs have been infiltrating the stratosphere since Midgley's invention, but only recently has the ozone layer started to erode. One reason for this is that the catalytic effect of the chlorine has been blocked by the presence of small amounts of nitrogen compounds in the stratosphere. But as the amount of chlorine accumulates with the increasing amounts of CFCs, the protective nitrogen compounds are overwhelmed and the chlorine starts destroying the ozone.

The scientists at the Snowmass conference noted that disappearance
of ozone over the Antarctic was slow at first, but in the ten year period
1977–87, 50 per cent of the winter ozone vanished.[20] That 50 per cent
figure may be higher. Michael Proffitt and colleagues of the National
Oceanic and Atmospheric Administration's laboratory in Boulder, Colorado refined the data further and say the loss is more like 75 per cent.
Moreover, ozone destruction is spreading in a ring reaching as far north
as the tip of South America where the loss of winter ozone is about 30
per cent.[21] These disturbing new findings stress the urgency of what the
Snowmass scientists concluded, that the stage is now set for explosive
destruction of the ozone shield over the rest of the world. It is a matter
of time. How much time?

The Montreal Protocol: Phasing Out CFCs

Political leaders and CFC users feel that there is a fair amount of time.
In September 1987, representatives of twenty-three countries and the
European Economic Community's twelve member nations met in Montreal, Canada, under the leadership of the United Nations Environmental
Program (UNEP) to discuss limiting production of CFCs. They proposed a treaty that in 1990 would freeze world production of CFCs at
1986 levels and by 1999 would cut production by 50 per cent. This
treaty, known as the Montreal Protocol, was out of date even before it
was proposed in 1987; six months later, at the Snowmass meeting, when
the awesome truth of the Antarctic ozone hole became evident, Peter
Usher of UNEP, who had shepherded the Montreal Protocol to its
conclusion, said: 'The Montreal Protocol is not sufficient to repair the
Antarctic ozone hole. The hole is occurring now with about 3 parts per
billion [ppb] of chlorine in the atmosphere. Under the protocol, the
concentration of chlorine will increase to 6 or 7 ppb.' Usher said that
only a total ban would repair the damage.[22]

  Joe Farman, a scientist with the British Antarctic Survey, which
discovered the ozone hole, seconded Usher's conclusion, saying that we
currently put CFCs into the atmosphere five times faster than natural
processes destroy them, which means that even with a 50 per cent cut
by 1999 the amount of CFCs in the stratosphere will still be increasing.
Part of the problem of preventing destruction of ozone is the longevity
of the CFCs. Farman said that if CFC emission stopped tomorrow, one
third of the CFCs would still be in the stratosphere 100 years from now.
Our industrial society, in effect, has set in motion a train of events that

will run its course for the next three to ten human generations no matter what we do today.

With wide recognition that the Montreal Protocol will not halt ozone destruction, there is a move towards taking stronger action. The Dupont Company, the largest manufacturer of CFCs, unilaterally announced in 1988 that it was ceasing production of CFCs by the year 2000. The company said that it hoped its action would spur other countries to ban CFCs totally.

Dupont's action was not wholly altruistic. The company had a lead in developing replacements for the CFCs, and suggested the replacements be phased in as the CFCs are phased out. The technical problem is not quite that simple, because Dupont's replacements are also CFCs. To explain: the current CFCs are what are called fully substituted. That is, the compounds contain no hydrogen. The Dupont replacements are partially substituted, which means they contain less chlorine and some hydrogen. These partially substituted CFCs[23] are still lethal to the ozone shield, but only about one twentieth as much. Critics say that all CFCs, both the fully substituted and the partial, should be banned. The partially substituted CFCs may be less damaging, but in view of the enormous volume of these substances that will be vented, they could in practice be as destructive as the fully substituted CFCs.

While planning to stop production of fully substituted CFCs eventually, Dupont does not want governments forcing phase-out too quickly. Archie Dunham, vice-president of Dupont, warned that governments must tailor their policies to suit the chemical industry, or the search for replacement chemicals will be delayed or stopped altogether.[24] Dunham said the industry needs assurances that government will not interfere with development and production of the partially substituted CFCs and other replacements. It did not want to go to the expense of producing the replacements only to have governments ban them a few years later.

Prime Minister Thatcher and President Bush seem to go along with the CFC industry. Both said they would go further than the Montreal Protocol and recommend banning the fully substituted CFCs completely by the year 2000, providing suitable replacements could be found.[25] So it would seem that the speed at which CFCs are phased out depends, not on the speed at which the ozone shield is being eroded, but, as Liz Cook of Friends of the Earth says, on 'the timetable the chemical industry has set for itself'. She added, 'it doesn't force technological innovation.'[26]

Dupont is spending about $30 million a year on its search for replacements; a tiny sum, considering the CFC industry was worth $8 billion in 1987. It is also tiny in comparison to what is spent on curative medicine: that $30 million would pay for only 0.5 per cent of all US heart bypass operations.

It is these kind of institutional contradictions that make resolution of even a straightforward cause-and-effect environmental problem take on a molasses-like stickiness. Michael McElroy, an atmospheric scientist and head of the Department of Earth and Planetary Sciences at Harvard University, told a conference sponsored by the Canadian Department of Environment in Toronto in June 1988 that if CFCs were not phased out in five years, the ozone layer would be destroyed. Whether or not the deadline is exactly five years, time is short; McElroy has a clear understanding of the resiliency principle, and what he is saying is that, although erosion so far seems slight, like the stone wall of a cathedral, the ozone shield may suddenly crumble.

10

Global Warming

'The commons' was a large pasture in old English villages that belonged to no one; it belonged to everyone. Each villager could graze his cows there as much as he wished, but if too many villagers grazed too many cows, the pasture was ruined for everyone. The world ecosystem is a commons shared by everyone and everything on the planet, and, like the village commons, no country owns a piece of it. The global commons remains the same size and, as with the village commons, individual nations and societies through individual actions risk over-using it. The village commons regenerated as long as it was not overstressed, and the global commons too regenerates – up to a point. We do not know what that point is, nor do we understand all the factors that stress the global commons. We know that fossil fuel combustion and the release of CFCs cause much stress, and we are now beginning to identify other factors, all of which merge into an overwhelming stress on the global commons. One symptom of this global stress that is now grabbing public attention is global warming.

Lewis Thomas, in his book *Lives of the Cell*,[1] pictured the world ecosystem as a gigantic organism governed by the same principles that govern the lives of all organisms. One of those principles is that each organism works best at a precise average temperature. For the world organism this optimum is 15°C. For humans it is 37°C, and you know that, if you have a fever, it is a symptom that something is not right. There can be many causes for the fever; you are just aware of the end result. Whatever the cause, a fever exacts its toll because the efficiency of body chemistry falls off as temperature rises, and unless the causes are corrected the fever itself can be fatal. Atmospheric scientists are now telling us that the world ecosystem is about to experience a fever: the average temperature of the world will rise by about 5°C to about 20°C, within the lifespan of today's teenagers. Can you imagine the state of your health if you had a fever of 42°C?

Global warming is not an easy concept to deal with in government bureaucracies and industry boardrooms. Chemical waste dumps and city garbage, although they may not be dealt with adequately, at least are visible forms of pollution, something you can get your hands on. But how do you get your hands on something vaguely called global warming, particularly when the warming is a symptom of multiple stresses on a global scale? It is apparent that we need to rethink radically the way we deal with environmental issues.

This point was made by Hans Martin, an atmospheric scientist with Canada's Department of Environment. He told a conference on the costs of protecting the environment that the economic system is dangerously out of date when it comes to dealing with the environment. 'We have been conquering nature for 200 years,' he said in interview; 'now we have to realize that we are heating it to death.' This beating is not intentional brutality: we beat nature to death by the mere fact of living. An English medieval villager could not stop his cows from eating and dropping their wastes: in fact, the cows' wastes were part of the regenerative cycle of the commons. But the commons could accommodate only a certain size of cow economy; beyond that size, the commons failed to regenerate and turned into a waste-strewn, muddy field. An overstressed village commons was obvious to the villagers, and they seemed able to adjust their collective use to prevent such a fate. The global commons is not so easy to see, much less a rallying point to gather all users into common agreement of how to prevent its death by beating. Nevertheless, nothing short of global remedies will do. 'All nations are tied together as to their common fate,' observed Peter Raven, director of the Missouri Botanical Garden and a specialist in global ecology, in an interview with *Time* magazine. He added: 'We are facing a common problem, which is, How are we going to keep this single resource we have, namely the world, viable?[3]

Serious thoughts, but, as Hans Martin says, we have a great deal of difficulty in translating such thoughts into appropriate action. In this book I have been building a case that to succeed in the translation we have to discard the outmoded thinking of our environmental institutions, which filter their view of the world through the one-cause/one-effect biomedical model whereby a specific environmental hazard is linked to a specific human health effect. Such an approach provides a measure of environmental protection, but as we shall see, with an issue on the scale of global warming the approach is too feeble. If global warming were the Wimbledon tennis champion, our corrective actions would amount to no more than a Saturday afternoon recreational player.

A Duck's View of the Viability of its Ecosystem

Is global warming really upon us, and if so, how is it making its presence known? Ask a duck about the summer of 1988. A duck's-eye view of the North American ecosystem that summer, the hottest ever recorded, shows what a few extra degrees does to duck ecology. Ducks like to breed in small water holes; but most of the ponds where they formerly nested had evaporated in the heat. The grassy vegetation around the few remaining ponds withered away, stripping the ducks of cover from their predators. So they congregated in large flocks at the larger lakes; but ducks need privacy when they mate and few pairs nested. Overall: a bad year for ducks. Wildlife specialists say it will take years for the duck population to recover from the dryness of the 1988 season, even assuming there are no more extraordinarily dry and hot summers in the next few years.

But the ducks *are* in for more bad summers, according to James Hansen, Director of the Goddard Institute for Space Studies, New York, who has said that global warming is not something that is going to happen in the next century; it has arrived. Scientists have been talking of global warming for a long time, but always in terms of a distant future. For most people, there was no sense of urgency or understanding of what a slight rise in average global temperature means to the individual. Hansen uses a pair of dice to illustrate what it means in terms of weather. One die represents the climate for the period 1950–80: two sides are white for normal summer temperatures, two sides are blue for colder-than-average summers and two sides are red for hotter-than-average summers. Thus on the roll of the die there are two chances out of six of having an extra hot summer. The situation, however, has changed. Hansen's second die represents the 1990s: one side is white, one is blue, and four sides are red. 'The greenhouse warming in the 1990s will be sufficient to shift the probabilities such that the chance of a hot summer in most of the country will be in the range of 55 to 80 percent,' he said. 'There will be more hot summers than normal, and the hottest ones will be hotter than they used to be.'[4]

The dice, Hansen emphasized, are loaded. What he meant was that once the warming trend starts it is not easily or quickly reversed. The reason can be found in what we call the greenhouse effect. Although news reports talk of the greenhouse effect as causing global warming, it is not a new happening. In fact, without it most of planet earth would look like the Antarctic. We need the greenhouse effect to maintain habitable temperatures. We all know that the sun's rays provide light and heat; but the earth captures the sun's heat in the same way as a greenhouse operates.

The Greenhouse Effect

The sun's rays are like a flying football: you only feel their force when they strike you. Similarly, sunlight travels the 155 million km (96 million miles) from the sun, passes through the atmosphere and gives off heat only when it strikes the earth's surface. Sunlight passes through the earth's atmosphere as visible light, but when the warmed-up earth radiates heat back it radiates it as infrared light. Now, if the atmosphere consisted only of oxygen and nitrogen, the energy received from the sun would, in effect, bounce right back into space as infrared light, and the average temperature of earth would be an iceball of $-25°C$. What makes life on earth possible is the presence in the atmosphere of what scientists call greenhouse gases, the main ones being water vapour, carbon dioxide and methane. These gases absorb much of the infrared light radiated from the earth's surface, in effect acting as a blanket to trap heat at the earth's surface. The result: planet earth has an average temperature of 15°C, suitable to sustain its life.

It is the same principle as that of the greenhouse: the sun's energy is trapped inside the house as heat, because, while the window glass is transparent to the incoming visible light, it blocks outward passage of the infrared rays. The greenhouse effect has always existed, but the problem today is that, while the greenhouse gases have held at a steady level in the earth's atmosphere since the last ice age, the amounts of some of them, notably carbon dioxide and methane, have risen slowly since the beginning of the industrial revolution. That rise has now accelerated to a gallop, and because there is more of these gases, they trap more of the earth's escaping heat. It is similar to putting a thicker blanket on your bed.

The threat of global warming was predicted as early as 100 years ago by the Swedish chemist, August Arrhenius (1859–1927). He pointed out that increased industrial activity would increase the amount of carbon dioxide in the atmosphere, and as a result of his prediction, scientists have been measuring the amounts of the greenhouse gases ever since. But they could not be sure when we would start to notice the warming;

climate by its nature is highly variable and local, and only by looking
back over a long period can one see a trend. The British shivered in the
summer of 1988, while the ducks and people of North America baked,
and in fact, according to Mick Kelly of the Climate Research Unit at
the University of East Anglia, a portion of northern Europe has cooled
by 0.25°C over the last twenty years.[5] He suggested that the closeness
of the sea may be a factor and that some parts of the world may indeed
show cooling while other parts, particularly large land masses like North
America, show a warming trend.

It may be another twenty years before warming on a global scale is
fully established, although James Hansen believes that the trend is now
apparent: '[There] is ample justification for my testimony,' he wrote in
a letter to the editor of the *New York Times*, 'that the greenhouse effect
is changing our climate now.'[6] Assuming Hansen is correct, what can
we look forward to? He and other atmospheric experts predict a 1.5–5°C
rise in global temperature at least by 2060 and perhaps by as early as
2030.[7] That means a young person entering the work force today will
retire in a much warmer world. That world's ecology will look very
different.

Whereas humans and other warm-blooded animals maintain constant
body temperature regardless of the outside temperature, a major fraction
of the world's life – insects, sea life, bacteria and plants – assume the
temperature of their environment. A major effect of global warming
will be on plants, because most plants grow best at a precise average
temperature. You do not find birch forests, for instance, on the Riviera
or in Alabama: they prefer the relatively cool summers and frigid winters
of the Soviet Union and Canada. Jag Maini, a senior forestry official in
the Canadian federal government, said that the trees being planted in
Canada's reforestation programme – trees adapted over thousands of
years to Canada's summers and winters – may not survive if the average
temperature goes up before they mature fifty years from now. 'The
change that we expect is beyond the evolutionary experience of these
trees,' he said.[8]

Could new strains of trees be developed that would survive a rise in
temperature? It is not that simple, and Maini was pessimistic. Because
of a tree's long growing period, he doubted whether scientists would be
able to adapt new strains of trees to changing and unpredictable climatic
conditions.

Climatic change is the norm for planet earth; the northern part of the
planet is only 18,000 years out of the last ice age. Life adapts. But
such natural swings in climate are unnoticeable on a human timescale,
occurring at a pace that gives trees and all other life forms opportunity

to adapt. It now looks as if human society is about to experience a major swing in global climate well within the lifespan of an individual. This pace of change is unprecedented, according to Michael McElroy, who says: 'It is this aspect of the problem that is most bothersome.'[9]

The Greenhouse Gases are Increasing

What prompts McElroy, Hansen, Maini and other scientists to make such gloomy predictions? Not all scientists agree with them, and indeed there is argument over if or when global warming will start and to what extent the temperature will rise. But there is no doubt that the amounts of the greenhouse gases are increasing. These are hard facts over which there is no dispute and which are the basis for the prediction. The earth is being covered, so to speak, by a thicker blanket.

Methane and carbon dioxide are produced naturally by living processes. Methane is a gas produced by bacterial decomposition of vegetation in the absence of oxygen, but although the process is natural, human activity greatly increases the amount of such decomposition. Cattle decompose vegetation in their stomachs, and the great herds of cattle in all parts of the world produce about 20 per cent of the total methane. Rice paddies, which provide half of the calories consumed by the earth's population, have vegetation that rots under water, producing methane instead of carbon dioxide. Methane is twenty-five times as effective as carbon dioxide in absorbing the infrared radiation, so decomposition of vegetation in cattle stomachs and rice paddies, by producing methane rather than carbon dioxide, is the equivalent of putting on a wool blanket instead of a cotton blanket.[10] The amount of methane in the atmosphere has doubled since pre-industrial times and is increasing by between 1 and 2 per cent a year.

Carbon dioxide is the largest single greenhouse gas, trapping about half the total heat. The atmospheric concentration of carbon dioxide from the last ice age to the beginning of the nineteenth century was 280 parts per million (ppm). But industrial activity added to the natural generation of carbon dioxide with the burning of the fossil fuels, coal and oil. The concentration of carbon dioxide rose to 315 ppm in 1958 and to 345 ppm in 1988, increasing by 1.5 ppm each year. At the present rate of increase in fossil fuel burning, the figure will reach 550 ppm by about 2060, a doubling over the concentration of the pre-industrial era.

The increase in amounts of carbon dioxide and methane is in itself sufficient to boost global temperature by as much as the predicted 5°C. But what is causing the scientists to talk of an unprecedented pace of change is the rapidly growing contribution of the man-made pollutants, ozone, nitrogen oxides and CFCs. Together these products of industrial society contribute almost as much to the greenhouse effect as carbon dioxide and methane.

Ozone and nitrogen oxides both trap infrared radiation. Ozone is generated at ground level by the action of sunlight on volatile pollutants in the air, such as gasoline vapour. Do not confuse this ozone with the ozone layer of the stratosphere; the world does not need this low altitude ozone. It not only traps infrared radiation, it corrodes buildings and poisons plant life. The nitrogen oxides, produced in motor vehicle engines and fossil fuel-fired electrical power plants, are a major compon-ent of acid rain and, it turns out, a major trapper of infrared radiation. Because of increasing industrial activity and the increasing number of cars and trucks on the road, the greenhouse effect of ozone and nitrogen oxides is expected to triple in the next thirty years.

The CFCs are more bad news. One of the ironies of the hot North American summer of 1988 was that factories worked overtime to supply 3.6 million new home air conditioners. The air conditioning units contain CFCs, all of which will someday enter the atmosphere. The CFCs absorb infrared light 20,000 times more effectively than carbon dioxide, and although the amount of the CFCs is smaller, their contribution is significant. By the year 2020, ozone, nitrogen oxides and CFCs, all products of the industrial lifestyle, will double the greenhouse effect from the level caused by increasing amounts of carbon dioxide and methane. It adds up to a pretty thick blanket.

Global Feedback

Although it is straightforward to describe global warming in terms of a greenhouse – the greenhouse gases being the window glass – this analogy is a grossly simplified one. The greenhouse metaphor conveys how the sun warms the earth, but it only partially conveys why the earth is starting to warm up. Many factors in addition to the greenhouse gases affect global warming. Some of these factors counterbalance the effect of a thicker layer of greenhouse gases; other factors accelerate the warm-ing. The factors are all part of an elaborate feedback mechanism that has stabilized world temperature at 15°C.

Feedback is critical in maintaining evenness of temperature. Your boiler thermostat is a feedback mechanism. When the room gets hotter the thermostat shuts down the boiler; when the room cools, the thermo-stat turns it back on. Overall, room temperature holds steady. Scientists know in general about feedback mechanisms in the world ecology, but they have not identified all of them, nor do they understand how all the mechanisms interact with one another. Cloud cover, for instance, can be a negative feedback. Global warming may increase cloud cover, which reflects more of the sun's energy before it reaches the earth. Some scientists believe that the increased cloud cover will be sufficient to cancel global warming. V. Ramanathan of the University of Chicago, who studies the effects of cloud cover, however, said in interview with the *New York Times* that it would be a dangerous mistake to assume that clouds will take care of the greenhouse effect: 'We still don't understand the balance and how clouds will respond to warming. That is a major uncertainty.'[11]

In the other direction, a positive feedback is the equivalent of pouring gasoline on a fire: the more the earth warms, the faster it warms. Ocean sediments, for instance, contain vast amounts of methane. When the oceans warm – as they inevitably must do with a rise in global temperature – this methane is driven into the atmosphere, trapping still more heat. Warmer water also absorbs less carbon dioxide, so more remains in the atmosphere. It is such positive feedback that troubles scientists the most. Wallace Broecker, a geochemist at Columbia University, determined that there were rapid and extreme changes in world climate 10,000–13,000 years ago caused by a sudden reorganization of the ocean–atmosphere system.[12] In Broecker's view, what this means is that the global thermostat is sensitive to breakdown when pushed too far. In simple language, the checks and balances that stabilize the earth's temperature can fail: in effect, the thermostat stops working and the boiler goes crazy.

Predicting the Future

Politicians want to know the precise effects of global warming so they can take countermeasures if these are deemed necessary. One prediction, for instance, is that the melting of the polar icecaps and the warming of the oceans (the water will expand) will raise the sea level by as much as 1.5 m (8 ft). Coastal cities, alarmed at this prospect, want to know when to apply for grants from the federal governments for building dykes. But the clarity of the scientists' predictions is no better than that of a cloudy crystal ball, according to Stephen Schneider, a climatologist at the National Center for Atmospheric Research, Boulder, Colorado. For although scientists can measure and predict accurately the thickness of the blanket made up of the greenhouse gases, they are unable to predict precisely the effects of that thickening blanket. 'There are going to be sizable effects, we know that much,' said Michael Schlesinger of Oregon State University, another climatologist who is trying to clear the crystal ball by modelling the effects of global warming.[13] But mathematical modelling is highly imperfect because climate, which depends not only on the atmosphere but on land masses and oceans, has a complexity beyond the calculations of humans and computers. Still, while admitting the imperfections in their models, the scientists say that those models at least show general trends and that as Schlesinger said, they are certain that global warming is on its way and there will be climatic changes.

Where does this leave government policy-makers? Will they be able to act on the broad trends or are they going to wait until detailed effects are noticeable and then attempt a cure? Waiting is dangerous because ecological decay becomes unstoppable. Stephen Schneider draws a similar conclusion to Wallace Broecker: 'Humans are altering the earth's surface and changing the atmosphere at such a rate that we have become a competitor with natural forces that maintain our climate. What is new is the potential irreversibility of the changes now taking place.'[14]

The Fragile Globe

While the politicians are deciding what to do about global warming, the concept itself is radically shifting the image people have of global ecology. The situation is like a large, active family in their house. Trash gets scattered about, the walls get splattered and the shower sprouts a green slime. Family members argue over how much time each should spend cleaning up. Some members tolerate filth better than others, making the argument more caustic. Nevertheless, the family gets on with its life. But now the structure of the house is threatened. The roof develops a big hole, the walls crack, the foundation sags and the boiler overheats. Suddenly the family realizes that it lives in a fragile home.

The point of the analogy is that the trash and filth were undermining the structure of the house all along. What the family sees now are signs of fragility. Our industrial lifestyle has all along been undermining the very structure of our earthly house – our global ecosystem – but now signs of structural weakness hitherto ignored are appearing, some of them more obvious than others. The global warming sign is literally banging on our collective heads. It is hard to ignore.

This new awareness changes our image of how governments should deal with environmental problems, from dealing with local pollution to dealing with global decay: or, more simply, from dealing with the problems after the fact to dealing with them before the fact. Environmental protection hitherto has been an add-on activity. Governments created departments or agencies of environment to oversee clean-up after the pollution had occurred, in effect to sweep the floor after it has been littered. This form of environmental protection offered governments the luxury of deciding whether to sweep or not to sweep, particularly when sweeping was costly or appeared to interfere with economic gain. The after-the-fact approach to global warming can only take the form of adaptive strategies – building dykes to stem ocean tides, bioengineering new crops. It is futile. As Stephen Schneider says, 'society does not have the resources to hedge against all possible negative future outcomes.' He adds, 'we are perturbing the environment at a faster rate than we can predict the consequences.'[15]

Thinning the Greenhouse Blanket

So how should governments respond to the idea of a fragile globe and its warming? There are three ways of dealing with global warming. First, ignore it. Kenneth Watt, an ecologist in the Department of Environmental Studies in the University of California at Davis, called the greenhouse effect 'the laugh of the century'.[16] Lester Lave, an economist at Carnegie-Mellon University, admitted that a change in climate is likely, but said that is all we really know. 'There is no way to justify spending tens of billions of dollars a year to prevent the greenhouse effect,' he said in interview.[17]

The second way is to deal with the symptoms, like taking a drug to lower blood pressure or cholesterol level. The city of Charleston, South Carolina, a coastal city, is in the midst of planning a new sewer system in which it will incorporate the eventuality of a rising sea. American agricultural colleges have launched dozens of projects to develop new crop plants resistant to hot, dry weather. Tony Hall, a plant physiologist at the University of California at Riverside, believes plant scientists must move quickly. 'We're talking about dramatic changes in the next 50 years. It's a short time. We will barely have enough time to make the changes in agriculture that we need.'[18]

Rising sea levels and drought have indeed been predicted, but as already mentioned, many scientists stress that the most serious effects are likely to be unexpected: not things you can spend fifty years planning for.

The third way of dealing with global warming is by going to the root sources, that is, attacking the major source of the problem: the greenhouse gases. There are those like Watt and Lave who believe that the scientific evidence for global warming is not solid enough to warrant action; but what if Hansen, McElroy, Schneider and many other atmospheric and earth scientists are right? And if global warming turns out to be a laugh, what is lost by cleaning up some existing environmental problems?

Half the problem is carbon dioxide, but this gas is not normally thought of as a pollutant: in fact, it is a necessary component of life's cycles. Plants convert carbon dioxide to their own substance, which animals eat as food and convert back to carbon dioxide. Superimposed on this biological cycle is a geological cycle: oceans dissolve vast quantities of carbon dioxide and some of this is deposited as limestone rock. The rocks are thrust upwards to the surface by subterranean rumblings where they erode returning the carbon to the biological cycle. And so it has gone for a billion years.

The carbon cycles are natural. What is not natural is the sudden rush of carbon dioxide into the atmosphere, faster than it can be absorbed either by growth of new vegetation or into the oceans. Since the industrial revolution humans have been converting two great reservoirs of carbon into carbon dioxide: fossil fuel and trees. The world's tree cover is rapidly disappearing. The last major forested areas of the planet – the tropics – are being destroyed at a rate, in Albert Gore's words, of a football field a second. In 1988, destruction of forests in Brazil and other tropical countries contributed 25 per cent of carbon dioxide emissions for that year.

The industrial countries of the earth's temperate zone are busily telling tropical countries to stop this destruction, but the same countries are busily converting the second reservoir, fossil fuel, to carbon dioxide. The United States, the world's largest consumer of energy, generates 87 per cent of its energy from the burning of fossil fuel: coal, natural gas and petroleum. (Almost 60 per cent of American electricity is generated by coal-fired power plants.) The American economy (and that of all other industrialized nations) in naked reality runs on fossil fuel.

George Woodwell, director of Wood's Hole Research Center, Wood's Hole, Massachusetts, said: 'Stabilizing the atmosphere and the temperature of the earth will require a reduction [of coal and oil] by at least 50 per cent below current use.'[19] In addition, Woodwell recommended cessation of tropical forest destruction and initiation of massive reforestation. Woodwell's basic idea puts the global commons into concrete terms: the world cannot generate more carbon dioxide than can be trapped by the oceans and new plant growth. The earth's carbon dioxide budget will have a definite ceiling.

And while industrialized nations ponder if or how to cut fuel consumption, developing countries want a piece of the high living standard that high energy consumption brings. China, for example, has set a goal of reaching a level of industrialization equivalent to that of Western countries, based in large part on coal-fired electric power. And in addition, if they achieve the living standards of Western countries, they will be driving 500 million cars. Thus, if the fossil-fuel-using nations of the world set a global ceiling – as Woodwell says they must – on the amount of such fuel that can be burned, there will have to be some give and take between the high and low consumers of fossil fuels. This idea is not impracticable, considering the international treaties that have been negotiated in the face of global threats, for example, the nuclear non-proliferation treaty and the Montreal Protocol to phase out CFCs.

But cutting back fossil fuel consumption treads on vested interests. Joseph Mullan, senior vice president for environmental affairs at the US National Coal Association, contended in an interview with the *New York Times* that the role played by coal in contributing to atmospheric carbon dioxide is still unknown. Besides, Mullan noted, some scientists believe the earth is moving towards a new ice age that could cancel out the greenhouse effect.[20]

The next ice age is not due for another 1,500 human generations, which seems a long wait. There are those, including US Secretary of State James Baker, who urge that the solution to the problem of global warming should be launched now, by Mullan's generation. Baker told a seventeen-nation group formed to deal with global warming 'that political ecology is ripe for action. Time will not make the problem go away.'[21]

How should countries go about reducing carbon dioxide emissions? 'The only solution you're really left with, in a pragmatic sense, is nuclear.' These are the words of Richard Slember, vice-president and general manager of Westinghouse's energy systems, a major manufacturer of nuclear reactors.[22] Slember's view is obviously coloured by his industrial position, but it is a view that the nuclear industry, long in a slump, is increasingly putting forth. If nuclear power does make a comeback, the financial fortunes of Westinghouse and other nuclear companies will skyrocket. Six thousand new nuclear power plants will be needed (there are at present 500 worldwide) according to Alvin Weinberg, formerly head of the Oak Ridge National Laboratories. Weinberg, an advocate of nuclear power, says this number will be able to maintain the world's current rate of energy consumption and at the same time reduce carbon dioxide emissions to the break-even point, at which the absorption of carbon dioxide by the plant life and oceans equals production of the gas.

Weinberg, well aware of the tendency of nuclear reactors occasionally to run amok, admits there would be a safety problem with 6,000 reactors operating in the world. We could expect a Chernobyl-type accident every 1.5 years, he said, if the reactors attained only the current level of safety. But he added that he is confident this will not happen because the industry will design reactors that can be 'run by idiots'.[23] All very well, but in his enthusiasm for this technical fix, Weinberg did not address the problem of disposing of the radioactive waste from 6,000 reactors.

Somewhere in between Mullan and Slember and Weinberg is an innovative approach taken by Applied Energy Services of Arlington, Virginia. They are building a coal-fired electric power plant in Uncasville, Connecticut, and as part of the cost of construction they will plant 52 million trees in Guatemala. The growth of the trees will absorb an equivalent amount of carbon dioxide to that generated by the power plant, estimated to be 15 million tons, over its forty-year lifespan.[24]

Much more needs to be done. A group of scientists and policymakers meeting at a conference convened by the Canadian Department of Environment in June 1988 were so alarmed by the rush of information about global decay that they said the Montreal Protocol (agreed to by twenty-four industrial nations six months earlier to cut production of CFCs by 50 per cent by 2000) was out of date. They would phase out fully substituted CFCs by 2000 and aim for a 20 per cent cut in carbon dioxide emission by 2005, with a longer-term goal of stabilizing emissions at 50 per cent of their 1988 levels.[25] The urgency of getting started on the reductions was underscored by Michael McElroy: 'We face an immediate and important challenge: to understand and predict the consequences of our actions and to bring this knowledge to bear so as to preserve the viability of this planet for ourselves and for generations yet unborn.'[26]

A Sense of Global Responsibility

But again we come back to the reality of the ingrained habits that our industrial society finds hard to shed. Government leaders have long believed that environmental action falls into Adam Smith's economic wastebin. Smith, the father of modern economics, lived in the simpler era of the eighteenth century when he dismissed the work of 'servants, churchmen, lawyers, players, buffoons, musicians and opera singers as unproductive of any value'.

Smith's definition of productive worth – although he may not have intended it thus – gave us an image of global ecology that has prevailed in government thinking and action ever since, and which opposes the image that environmentalists are trying to get across to government leaders. Environmentalists see the world as a finite commons, capable of sustaining a vigorous and satisfying life as long as we adapt our human affairs to its limits. Economists, the modern disciples of Smith, see the world as kind of an inflatable globe, infinitely expandable with unlimited resources and with unlimited oceans and air in which to discard wastes. It is an appealing image; and it is the economists who receive Nobel Prizes and who are much admired in business and government circles, and it is the economists' image of the world that has prevailed. It is a reckless, sledgehammer view, however, one that in Albert Gore's words lacks a future: 'We transform the resources of the past into the pollution of the future, telescoping time for self indulgence in the present.'[27]

But suddenly in 1988, with the publicity given to global warming, the environmentalists' view of the world has started to make some inroads in economic and business thinking. Possibly economics and ecology will come closer together. Ironically, both words derive from the same Greek root: *oikos* means house or home. Ecology is the study or science of our earthly home – or we could say the study of the global commons and how it works. Economics refers to management of the home. The two aspects dovetail because such management should not be doing what Gore and many others say it is doing, destroying our earthly home.

It remains to be seen how fast and how far ecological thinking penetrates economic circles, how far government and business leaders are prepared to go in meeting Michael McElroy's challenge for 'a new sense of global responsibility'. Even if (or when) business and government leaders adopt a new responsibility, it is one thing to talk about it and another to translate it into action. There is a need for overall policy leadership and that can only come from central governments. So far, global warming and the greenhouse effect have been treated as a technical problem, something for scientists to wrestle with and come up with technical solutions for. It is not treated as an issue concerning the way we live our industrial lifestyle and as a need to adjust that lifestyle.

The problem of adjustment is not purely technical; it is economic, political and social. How easy is it to approach the issue in that light? Many scientists are pessimistic about the prospects for marrying up the technical and social aspects of the problem. James Friend, an atmospheric scientist at Drexel University, Philadelphia, said, 'I don't see how our current sociopolitical or economic systems can solve the greenhouse problem.'[28]

What is needed are new institutional arrangements; that is, we need to think about the social and political structures within which we try to grapple with these global problems. For instance, governments did not bring the environment into their structures in a formal way until the late 1960s or early 1970s, when they created departments or agencies of environment. All these departments, however, were designed for the add-on approach; their activities are supposed to correct environmental problems after they arise. The new awareness of global warming and global decay is beyond the add-on approach. It is obsolete. But can these bureaucratic units designated by their governments to deal with environmental issues switch to a preventive approach? Prevention cuts across the complete spectrum of government and social activity. Perhaps these separate departments and agencies should be abolished and the environmental function built into all government departments, with each taking an ecological responsibility. However it is done, it is clear that present departments of environment are not suited to dealing with the global commons.

Prevention concerns more than government departments: the ultimate success of environmental programmes depends on the public. Some officials are sceptical of human ability to make the broad adjustments necessary. William Ruckelshaus, a former head of EPA, said in a kind of despair: 'We are a long way in this country from taking individual responsibility for the environmental problem. Just drive down the highway and watch the guy in front of you throw junk out of his car window. Unless we can get individuals to act differently than they do now, we have a hell of a problem.'[29] What disturbs Ruckelshaus and other government officials is that people look for the quick fix, do anything except change their accustomed practices. One cannot help noting the parallel with personal health: pills, high-tech medicine, are looked upon as the solution to health problems. Or, if people become health-conscious, they eat a bran muffin as a way of cancelling the artery-clogging effect of a high-steak diet. But as noted in earlier chapters, this attitude is highly conditioned by the health-care system, and it is fair to suggest that if the health-care system were to foster true prevention (not just promotion), the public would be much more amenable to thinking about the global commons in preventive terms.

11

The Great Lakes Ecosystem

Only 250–400 white whales, the belugas, swim the lower St Lawrence River, where seventy five years ago 5,000 swam. These small members of the whale family – the largest male weighs about 1,000 kg (2,200 lb) – frequent inshore areas and are subject to more man-made pollution than their offshore relatives. The current population is mostly adult, because few young belugas are surviving. And, moreover, the adults are dying at about fifteen years of age, in human terms a young thirty-five. They die mainly of ordinary bacterial infections of the blood, which they are unable to resist because their immune system is depressed. Their carcasses, when they wash up on the shore, have to be carted away by men wearing protective clothing and be deposited in a hazardous waste dump. Belugas, in the words of Leone Pippard, a consultant to Parks Canada who studies the whales, are 'living garbage bins'.[1]

The St Lawrence is one of North America's mightiest rivers, the only outlet to the ocean for the Great Lakes system. This ecosystem of five massive lakes and connecting rivers extends almost to the centre of the continent, straddling the border between the United States and Canada. Within and around that basin, the Great Lakes hold one fifth of the world's fresh water, two fifths of all United States industry, one half of all Canadian industry and 40 million people. The people and their industries generate 100 million metric tons (110 million tons) of waste per year, which the Great Lakes basin, like a giant bathtub, collects and drains into the St Lawrence. The belugas, in effect, live in the drainpipe.

The belugas are only one sympton of ecosystem stress on the Great Lakes and the federal governments of both countries in recognition of this stress signed in 1978 a Great Lakes Water Quality Agreement.[2] The agreement launched a grand strategy to relieve all ecological stress, called an 'ecosystem approach'. The idea is to avoid dealing with problems on a piecemeal basis, mounting instead a co-ordinated attack. If the plan is successful it could serve as model of how to organize a comprehensive environmental clean-up in other parts of the two countries.

The ecosystem approach is of particular interest to our exploration of environmental thinking because it seems to go beyond the one-cause/one-effect approach. Could it be the preventive approach, the new wave of environmental protection that the Brundtland Commission so earnestly seeks? We shall see.

The environmental problems of the Great Lakes basin faced by the two countries are not simple. According to a joint study by the US National Academy of Sciences and the Canadian Royal Society, belugas and the human population in the Great Lakes basin are more exposed to toxic chemicals than those anywhere else in North America.[3] The major environmental issue in the Great Lakes basin, in fact, is toxic chemicals, and the ecosystem approach is really designed to eliminate the impact of these contaminants.

The Great Lakes Ecosystem: Is it Healthy?

The Great Lakes have a long history of urban and industrial activity. The major American cities of Buffalo, Cleveland, Detroit, Chicago, Milwaukee and Duluth, and the Canadian cities of Thunder Bay, Windsor, Hamilton, Toronto, Kingston and Montreal have grown steadily on this inland waterway. But until the Second World War, the size of the human population and its accumulated wastes had not seriously overloaded the ecosystem. Thirsty pleasure boaters could reach over the side and collect a glass of water to drink, an act unthinkable now. Since the war, population growth and industrial activity have shot up. Production and use of chemicals around the lakes alone has increased 63-fold. The Great Lakes ecosystem, of course, has not grown; it has not changed geologically since 4,000 years ago when a northern river to the Atlantic Ocean was sealed off, leaving the St Lawrence River as the sole drain.

If the five Great Lakes were people, they would have to be hospitalized, their webs of life in disarray. It is the study of wildlife, in fact, that reveals the precarious state of the lakes' ecology. The effects of chemical pollution are devastating.

Tumours are common, for example, in those fish living near lake cities where pollution is heaviest. John Harshbarger, director of the registry

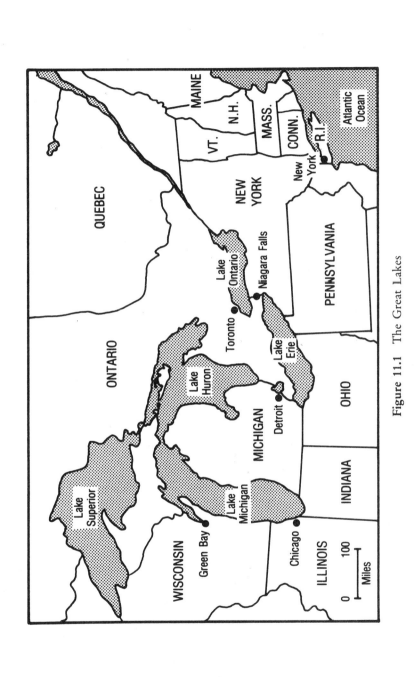

Figure 11.1 The Great Lakes

of tumours in lower animals at the National Museum of Natural History, said that all but one of fish tumour outbreaks that he was aware of occurred in areas of obvious pollution.[4] The tumours occur in the liver, the organ where foreign chemicals accumulate. Harshbarger said that before 1964 liver tumours were completely unknown in wild animals.

A variety of other ailments afflict the watery inhabitants. Coho salmon of Lake Erie, one of the most popular sports fish, suffer almost a 100 per cent incidence of goitre, which can be caused by chemical contaminants. The body chemistry of the coho, in fact, seems to be knocked awry: the fish have impaired fat metabolism, and many fish lack secondary sex characteristics; 75 per cent of coho embryos die.

Coho salmon are predatory fish, already far up the food chain. The toxic chemicals in the water are biomagnified two to ten thousand times in their flesh. Fish-eating birds magnify the chemicals another hundred fold. The double-crested cormorants of Lake Michigan are prone to a devastating teratogenic defect, not noticed before 1979. The birds hatch with crossed bills (like an open pair of scissors) that make it difficult for them to catch fish, and they die at an early age. James Ludwig, Ecological Research Services, Bay City Michigan, who studies the cormorants, tied the defect to chemical pollution. 'All waters of Lake Huron and Lake Michigan are still significantly contaminated,' he said.[5]

Toxic effects on wildlife can be subtle. Glen Fox, a biologist with the Canadian Wildlife Service, walks into herring gull colonies during nesting time when the birds resent intruders. Fox said when he went into one colony situated in an area relatively uncontaminated, 856 gulls swooped down at him and thirty-four violently struck his hard hat. When he went among a similar size colony on the shore of Lake Ontario, only thirty-four birds swooped at him, with one actual contact. 'They are not as aggressive as normal gulls,' he said. As a result, Fox added, the birds do not protect their nests and fail to incubate or raise their chicks properly.[6] An explanation for the gulls' wimpish behaviour comes from the studies of Michael Fry, a biologist at the University of California at Davis. He injected gull eggs with an amount of DDT equivalent to that of contaminated eggs in the wild. DDT interferes with imprinting of the embryo. A word of explanation. Hormonal changes occur at a specific point in male embryonic development, including that of humans, which imprints maleness. DDT blocks this hormonal imprinting. When the birds matured, Fry noted permanent suppression of strutting, crowing and vigorous mating behaviour.[7] In other words, exposure to DDT at a brief moment in embryonic development turned the males into wimps.

Suppression of maleness is not confined to birds. Helen Daly, a psychologist at the State University of New York, Oswego, fed rats on coho salmon caught in Lake Ontario. She said the rats became sluggish and emotionally fragile compared to control rats fed coho from the Pacific Ocean. The rats eating Lake Ontario coho were more afraid to seek food after receiving a mild electric shock, while the rats fed Pacific coho did not let a little shock stop them. Lake coho have a higher level of toxic chemicals than the ocean fish. Could eating toxic lake fish have similar effects on humans? Daly said she would like to study behavioural changes in humans. In any event, she personally was not taking chances. 'I know this,' she was quoted as saying, 'I will not eat fish from Lake Ontario.'[8]

The study of wildlife is becoming more sophisticated and revealing. At one time, scientists simply wanted to know if pollution killed wild animals. The level of pollution to do this has to be fairly high, usually from an episode like a chemical spill. But the behavioural studies detect adverse effects in animals chronically exposed to low levels of chemical contaminants. A casual glance shows the wildlife surviving, but what seem to be small changes in behaviour may in the long run threaten the existence of whole species.

Knowledge of Health Effects on Humans is Scanty

Scanty knowledge of the effects of environmental contaminants on human behaviour is one of the ongoing paradoxes of our environmental predicament. I have frequently raised the point that, while threats to human health drive environmental action, efforts to describe these threats in detail have been patchy and certainly unsystematic. The medical community, from lack of training and experience, is not set up to recognize clinical problems arising from environmental exposure. Doctors are more accustomed to seeing illnesses in the workplace: exposures are high and the effects fit into recognized clinical categories such as cancer, liver damage, neurological defects. Moreover, in the work place chemical exposure is easily connected to the illness. But no such connection arises with environmental exposure. The doctor faced with a sick person sees only a sick person.

And then there is the question of the next generation. Could teratogenic and imprinting effects noticed in lake animals show up in humans? The reproductive systems of animals are among the organs most easily damaged by small amounts of chemicals. Studying the damage in humans is difficult because of the long time we take to mature – most lake animals mature within a year or so. Nevertheless, a group of psychologists has developed innovative ways of studying adverse effects on infants born to mothers exposed to chemicals in their environment, and, as in the studies done on North Carolina infants mentioned earlier, the small amounts of chemicals are found sufficient to brake normal development.

Such studies require comparison of two groups, one with more exposure, one with less exposure. Harold Humphrey, an epidemiologist at the Michigan Department of Public Health, did the spadework to establish the two groups. He found that individuals who ate lake fish, which are contaminated with PCBs, DDT, dioxin and dozens of other toxics, had a higher level of such chemicals in their blood and body tissues compared to non-fish eaters.[9] There appeared, however, to be no difference in health patterns between the two groups, at least among the adults: the differences showed up in their children.

Three child psychologists, Greta Fein of the University of Maryland and a husband and wife team of Sandra and Joseph Jacobson from Wayne State University, Detroit, compared babies born to parents of the two groups and found that babies born to fish-eating mothers (higher exposure to the toxic chemicals) were 160–190 g (6–7 oz) lighter at birth and their head circumference was disproportionately smaller in relation to both birth-weight and gestational age (indicative of brain development). It should be noted that the chemicals in the mother's blood transfer through the placenta to the developing fetus, so the harm happens at some stage during fetal growth.

These researchers next examined the infants at six months old and found defects in visual recognition of the babies born to fish-eating mothers compared to the control group.[10] The memory defects were not noticed at birth; that is, the adverse effect is delayed.[11] The researchers wonder what other defects may show up later in life, a question they plan to study as the children grow up.

The Michigan study points up three flaws in the health-care system's policy towards adverse health effects of exposure to toxic chemicals. First, the medical community, all the while saying there is no evidence of harm from toxic chemicals in the Great Lakes basin, promotes few studies that could turn up such evidence: the big money goes to research on curing diseases. The Great Lakes fish-eater study is a rare event; consequently there is only a very tiny data base for assessment of human health effects.

The second flaw is that assessment is based on how medical doctors think in terms of clinical disease - something they are able to diagnose in their surgeries. Sub-clinical problems, such as memory recognition, do not come to their attention and tend to be excluded from the health-care system. Also doctors, guided by the biomedical model, prefer to think in terms of single causes, whereas environmental impacts can be multiple and delayed.

The third flaw is that when such studies are done, they are viewed in an isolated context. That is, if eating fish can be proven harmful the recommended solution, at least for prospective mothers, is to stop eating fish. The medical community is poor at putting together a broad picture from a variety of pieces of evidence. Consequently the public health significance of the Michigan study is lost. The families serving as a control group have about the same level of toxic contaminants in their bodies as all 40 million inhabitants of the Great Lakes region. It would be a mistake to assume that the level of contamination of a fish-eater must be reached before harm to fetuses and infants occurs. Any level of contamination causes stress to body tissues. It is a stress that, added to the other stresses of life, may or may not hasten a serious disorder – not only depressed mental capacity, but infertility or cancer.

A fourth flaw could be added: an unwillingness on the part of health authorities to incorporate data from wildlife studies. Information about the toxic damage to wild animals in the Great Lakes basin has been accumulating since the mid-1960s. Yet this type of information, twenty-five years later, is just not plugged into the experience and policy-making of the health-care system. There seems to be an assumption that the biology of human beings is different from that of other animals. If male seagulls are wimps – so much the worse for the seagulls.

In short, the professionals of the health-care system lack the intellectual framework in which to incorporate present information about environmental impacts on other species – and on humans – and to act upon this information. Their attitudes can be summed up by the remark of one doctor, a clinical toxicologist, at a meeting on health impacts of environmental chemicals, who said that he told his patients who asked about the effects of chemicals in their drinking water and residues in their food that there is no evidence whatsoever that such chemicals, at the exposure levels found in food and drink, can harm them.

Niagara Falls Dumps

Although governments talk of the ecosystem approach and its broad way of dealing with environmental issues, the crunch comes when action to clean up the pollution is undertaken. We will now look at one source of lake pollution and the plans to deal with it. The source is literally under the feet of millions of tourists who come every year to Niagara

Falls, NY. Eight million metric tons of highly toxic chemical waste lies buried under the city within walking distance of the famous falls. This waste is a legacy of the chemical industry, which, attracted by cheap electrical power in the latter part of the last century, established itself in Niagara Falls. The manufacture of chemicals generates vast quantities of toxic waste, and for 100 years the industry disposed of its wastes in the cheapest way possible: by pouring them into the Niagara River or burying them in one of 215 dumps. The most notorious of the 215 is Love Canal, but it is by no means the worst.

The 63-fold increase in the chemical production of North America since the end of the Second World War is fully reflected at Niagara Falls. The river and land area, however, has not grown 63-fold. It is like an outdoor privy designed to accommodate one person that must now accommodate 63. Not surprisingly, toxic overflow became apparent. But it was not until the 1970s that State and federal governments acknowledged that dumping might present an environmental hazard.

The types of chemicals buried in the dumps – PCBs, dioxin, DDT and hundreds of different chlorinated organics – are the most toxic of all man-made chemicals and the most persistent. They have the potential of poisoning the world biosphere for centuries. Douglas Hallett, a biologist with Canada's Department of Environment, has said that one shovelful of the gunk from one of the dumps is sufficient to poison all the wildlife of Lake Ontario.

The story of the government's clean-up plan for the 215 toxic waste dumps can be summed up in the story of one of them, located on the factory site of Occidental Chemical Corporation (formerly Hooker Chemical Co.). Its chemical factory is strung along the bank of the Niagara River about 5 km (3 miles) above the falls. The dump, officially called the 'S' Area Landfill, is situated 200 m (600 ft) from the edge of the river. Occidental began dumping toxic waste at this site in 1961, but its existence was known only to company officials, remaining hidden from the public until a bizarre incident took place.

The city of Niagara Falls had built its water treatment plant next to the Occidental Chemicals plant. Water is drawn through a long tunnel that runs under the river to the river's midpoint where the water intake is located. In 1978, water flow began to diminish, and the city engineers sent a team of scuba divers into the tunnel to find out what was wrong. The divers found that a heavy, sticky rubble had broken into the tunnel and partially blocked water flow. When brought to the surface, the rubble reeked of chemicals, and where it had splashed on to the divers' wetsuits, the fabric had disintegrated. Chemical analysis of the rubble revealed a mix of toxic chemicals of the type manufactured by Occidental.

Officials of the company at first denied that their chemicals could be leaking into the tunnel, and the city itself sought to reassure the public. The city manager said he was satisfied the drinking water was 'totally safe'. It was only after prodding from New York State investigators and EPA officials that Occidental Chemicals revealed the existence of the 'S' Area Landfill. If toxic wastes from this dump were infiltrating the city water intake, they were clearly spreading through the rock strata and reaching Niagara River.

The bedrock is not solid; it is fractured both horizontally and vertically, which means fissures run through it in all directions. A Canadian hydrogeologist, Grant Anderson, who studied the rock formation in this area, said that the contents of the dump could ooze down through the rock into the groundwater and into the river. Niagara River conveys the full flood of water from Lake Erie to Lake Ontario, a distance of about 50 km (30 miles), with the falls situated about 20 km (12 miles) from where it empties into Lake Ontario. Thus any pollutant that contaminates the Niagara River ends up in Lake Ontario. Canada's major cities and industrial activity are located on the shores of Lake Ontario, and some 4 million Canadians obtain their drinking water from the lake. Canada, therefore, has as much interest in cleaning up the dumps as the United States.

It was in the late 1970s that the public became alarmed over the dumps, but the United States, with the jurisdiction, seemed in no hurry to sponsor a clean-up. The EPA, the responsible federal agency, assigned to the issue a small staff headed by Michael Elder, who decided that rather than deal with all 215 dumps he would deal with the worst of them, which included the Occidental Chemicals 'S' Area Landfill. Occidental Chemicals had no intention of doing anything about the dump on its own initiative: in fact, the company maintained that the dump posed no threat to anyone. The only way for EPA to force action was to sue.

Although the existence of and problem with the 'S' Area dump came to light in 1978, Elder was already busy suing Occidental Chemicals over another of its dumps. He could handle only one dump at a time, so he did not get around to the 'S' Area dump until 1982, four years later. In order to bring the case to court, Elder had to squeeze the environmental problem into the structure of the law, and here is where law and biomedical model merge. The law states that it is necessary to connect the chemicals in the dump to evidence of actual harm or the potential for harm to humans. Wildlife does not count. Therefore, Elder had to build a legal case on evidence of harm to humans.

Although Canada had the greatest stake in the outcome of the suit, the Canadian government backed off the case; it did not want to be directly involved. Instead, it provided a citizens' group with expert help and a grant to pay court costs. The government itself was not prepared to put its prestige and power on the line, preferring to let the citizens' group enter the legal fray and take the blame if things did not go well – which they didn't.

The citizens' group wanted to be a fully fledged participant in the lawsuit with access to all documents and the right to cross-examine Michael Elder and representatives of Occidental Chemicals. The case came before Judge John Curtin of the United States District Court, Buffalo, NY. Before the Canadians would be allowed to participate (the legal term is 'intervenor' status), they had to prove to Curtin three propositions: (1) that chemicals in the 'S' Area Landfill were toxic; (2) that chemicals from this dump were leaking into the Niagara River; and (3) that the Canadian petitioners drank the water from downstream and were actually harmed by chemicals from the 'S' Area Landfill.

It was no secret that the Canadian group, if granted the right to participate in the suit against Occidental Chemicals, would press for destruction of the chemicals in the landfill. There are techniques for destroying chemical waste developed by Dutch engineers which involve incineration of the waste in a rotary kiln. The estimated cost for destroying the chemicals in the 'S' Area Landfill was $100 million. The EPA, however, pressed for a much cheaper remedy: building a concrete retaining wall around the dump. Occidental Chemicals, seeing a $100 million invoice before them, not surprisingly opposed the participation of the Canadians, and hired experts to prove their petition to obtain intervenor status had no merit.

One of these experts, Andrew Sivak of Arthur D. Little Inc., a Boston consulting company, undermined the Canadians' petition with the argument that the chemicals in the dump are indeed toxic, but at the levels found in drinking water are harmless. He then pointed to the discharge of chemicals from the 215 dump sites, not to mention nineteen municipal and industrial waste pipes. How then, he asked, could the Canadian groups claim they were being harmed by chemicals from the 'S' Area Landfill when the water was also contaminated from all these other sources?

Sivak's argument was based on the narrowest interpretation of the biomedical model: that is, it must be proven that a particular chemical from a particular source causes a clinical illness in an exposed person. How could such proof ever be obtained? Sivak knew very well such proof is unobtainable, but that aspect of the science was inadmissible in the court. In other words, the court had no legal framework to accommodate an ecosystem approach. The body of law had no way of acknowledging that there is a constellation of toxic chemicals in the environment, from many sources, all mixing together into one soup, and that everyone is exposed to the soup. The harm that arises is from the soup, not a single chemical from a single dump.

Judge Curtin, whatever his personal feelings, said, 'My job is to interpret the law.' He accepted the contention of Occidental Chemicals' hired geologists that the toxic chemicals were not migrating in the bedrock, he dismissed evidence of current and future ecological damage as irrelevant, and he threw out the Canadian petition for intervenor status.[12] This left the EPA and Occidental Chemicals to negotiate; they agreed – with the blessing of Judge Curtin – that the company would build the concrete retaining wall, costing some $15 million, around the 'S' Area Landfill. It is a short-term solution in which surface runoff is collected, but the toxic contents remain; and moreover, the bottom of the dump remains open with the possibility that, because the rock strata tilts, the contents will eventually slide under the retaining wall through the bedrock into the river.

With every passing year the solution of the 215 Niagara toxic waste dumps becomes more difficult and expensive. Like molasses on a sponge, the more the contents of the dumps spread through the underlying bedrock, the more rock there is to dig up. Nevertheless, the job can be done. The barrier to cleaning up the Niagara Falls' dumps is not technical, nor is it financial – compare a total bill of about $21 billion for the 215 dumps to the $50 billion or so a year the residents of the State of New York spend on health care – rather, it is lack of resolve and lack of a vision of how the ecosystem really works.

It is easy for the political leaders of Canada and the United States to announce that they are going to apply the ecosystem approach, but the political leaders at the same time have not created a legislative framework that takes into account the existence of a 'chemical soup'. Their plan to deal with pollution in a broad way cannot work when it remains chained to a set of old laws and legal attitudes.

The Ecosystem Approach at Work?

Although the Niagara Falls dumps are not the proudest example of the ecosystem approach, in all fairness the approach is being applied to diverse pollution problems within a local area. Forty-two areas of the

Great Lakes have been designated environmental hot spots, areas that are particularly dirty, such as harbours and estuaries, and Niagara Falls and its dumps are one of the forty-two. In bureaucratic parlance, the hot spots are allocated Remedial Action Plans (RAPs). One of them is Green Bay.

Green Bay is a large bay in Lake Michigan which slices like a sabre into the State of Wisconsin north of Chicago. The bay is 193 km (120 miles) long and about 22 km (14 miles) wide, with an average depth of 16 m (52 ft). The bay, with its surrounding towns, industries and farmlands, represents a distinct area that we can call the Green Bay ecosystem. It is an ecosystem severely stressed: the bay is a sink for all the sins of environmental mismanagement – inadequately treated sewage, farm runoff, soil erosion, destruction of wetlands, and industrial waste from the largest concentration of pulp and paper mills anywhere in the world.

The Green Bay RAP, on paper, has three notable features: it asks how the human economy can be modified so as to restore and sustain the local ecosystem; it takes an ecosystem approach by looking at the total picture; and it involves the local people in the decision-making. The RAP started rolling in the early 1980s, guided by the Great Lakes Fisheries Commission which took on the role of co-ordinator.[13] It would be nice to report that this rehabilitation programme was proceeding smartly, but some eight years later the RAP is stalled on the launch pad. This is no reflection on the plan's merits: rather, it reflects the difficulties of hurdling bureaucratic barriers, the difficulty of dealing with the mindsets of fragmented jurisdictions.

The agricultural community, for instance, is a major contributor to the bay's destruction. Rich dairy farms occupy about two thirds of the watershed, and the runoff unimpeded by woodlands carries huge amounts of eroding topsoil, fertilizers and chemical pesticides into the bay. The runoff is a byproduct of the farmers' practice of chemical-intensive agriculture. It is the only kind encouraged by government departments of agriculture and the agribusiness infrastructure. To switch the style of farming to an ecologically sound style that avoids soil erosion and fertilizer and pesticide runoff requires a change in the mindset of agricultural departments, a change which, as noted earlier, is blocked by the powerful vested interests of chemical agriculture. Any relief of this environmental stress on the bay thus strikes at the heart of current agricultural practice. Only if the move to sustainable (organic) agriculture gathers steam is there hope of reducing the chemical stress. But this factor lies outside the RAP, which illustrates just how limited a force it is in practice.

Jurisdictional fragmentation rather than co-ordination is another reality of local politics. The Green Bay watershed is administered by twenty-four counties as well as the fragmented bureaucracies of federal and State governments. The counties have the budgets and authority to control development and launch actions that affect the bay. But you will not find line items in these budgets with the financial dimensions to put the RAP in motion. You are asking a local councilman with a fixed budget to choose between buying a bulldozer and spending money on some environmental remedy that does not appear to offer the immediate benefit the bulldozer does. Neither the State of Wisconsin nor the federal government seems prepared to create a superbody with the deep pockets and the authority to move the plan ahead. The Great Lakes Fisheries Commission, with its overall co-ordinating responsibility, is an advisory body unarmed with either political clout or funds.

The Green Bay RAP in its grandest sense is prevention; it is a means to redesign personal, community and industrial lifestyle so that they blend in with the local ecology. But somehow the idea has got side-tracked, because in setting up the RAP no attempt was made to organize the institutional arrangements – the political and bureaucratic jurisdictions and powers. They remain fragmented and uncertain how to act. As William Reilly, head of the EPA, said, we talk of bold plans to protect the environment, but we fail to provide the organizational framework within which to be bold.

Long-range Transport of Pollutants

The ecosystem approach with its RAPs is an honest attempt to solve environmental problems at a local level, and there is no doubt that there are serious local problems to be solved. But environmental problems are like those Russian wooden dolls, stacked one inside another, and the Great Lakes ecosystem is stacked inside a continental ecosystem that is stacked inside a world ecosystem. If all forty-two RAPs were wildly successful, the 215 Niagara dumps were cleaned up and municipal and industrial waste and farm runoff was stopped, the pollution of the Great Lakes would still be serious. As much as 50 per cent of the toxic pollution entering the Great Lakes basic comes via long-range transport of pollutants from distant places, beyond the jurisdiction of the RAPs.

Most toxic chemicals are volatile, and whenever they are exposed to air they slowly evaporate. The handling of toxic wastes in hundreds of thousands of different places, often carelessly, means that these substances are spread over much of the North American landscape, and just as a thin film of water on the floor evaporates, so too the chemicals evaporate. Collecting toxic waste for disposal does not always provide control. The chemicals can evaporate from landfill, or if the waste is incinerated, poor incinerator design can lead to the toxic chemicals shooting unburned straight into the air. These air-borne chemicals are eventually washed out of the air, often thousands of kilometres from where they started. The Arctic pollution mentioned earlier, is the result of long-range transport. The Great Lakes, because of their huge water-shed, also collect a large fallout of this airborne filth. The chemical fallout is poorly recognized in environmental legislation for two reasons: the law needs a defined source to assign blame or designate control – how do you control rainfall or air currents? – and long-range transport gives chemical pollutants ample opportunity to migrate freely between land, air and water. The laws, to facilitate the work of Judge Curtin and other law administrators, partition the environment into what they call media: land, air and water. The partitioning is a superficial attempt to facilitate control, but it makes no sense. For example, acid rain starts out as an air pollution problem; it then becomes a water and land pollution problem – but government regulation can only be applied to the air. Different sets of regulations for the different media lead to contradicitions. A toxic chemical may be regulated in water but not in the air or vice versa. A factory faced with a stringent water emission regulation, can shoot the toxic chemical up the plant smokestack unregulated. Environmental policy-makers now talk of cross-media laws and regulations in which a pollutant will be tracked and controlled in all media simultaneously. This kind of thinking, however, in most countries has yet to be translated into actual practice.

Judge Curtin's decision regarding a remedy for the 'S' Area Landfill was made on the basis of a single medium, the land. How do you apportion blame for pollution when chemicals travelling from distant and multiple sources mix and interact with each other? It is impossible to identify any one source. In effect, such pollution remains above the law.

In Search of Lasting Solutions

Long-range transport evokes such words as multiple, cross-media, mixing, chemical soup. Yet when the Canadian and United States governments signed their Water Quality Agreement of 1978 (note the agreement addresses a single medium – water), they acted as if such terms did not exist in their vocabulary; they based their whole strategy for environmental clean-up on control of chemicals one at a time. Their so-called ecosystem approach shrinks to identification of a small number of designated toxic chemicals and the control of each. Can this lead to environmental clean-up?

In fact, what does environmental clean-up mean? Does it mean clean-up of all chemicals? The governments' definition of clean-up under the Water Quality Agreement actually means clean-up of only 350 toxic chemicals. Moreover, the official list shortlists eleven for critical attention. The list seems fly-size in comparison to the elephant-size list of manufactured chemicals actually used in the Great Lakes basin – about 60,000. About 50,000 of these have never been tested for their toxicity, and the 350 are selected from the 10,000 for which there is some information about harm. What of the other 50,000? Even for the 10,000, information is less than scanty; a survey by the US Academy of Sciences found that the number of manufactured chemicals for which there is extensive knowledge of environmental toxicity is nil.[14] In other words, how do you select 350 chemicals out of the soup when the data base for the selection is almost non-existent? Under the circumstances, the sensible thing would be to assume that all the chemicals are toxic.

Thus, when you probe the governments' idea of an ecosystem approach, you find a lot of outmoded baggage, the kind of beliefs about environmental problems common in the 1960s: the belief that a chemical is harmless until proof of its harm holds up in a court of law; the belief that each chemical must be judged alone (the concept of mixing, synergy, multiple insults is left out); the belief that pollution always comes out of the end of a pipe or smokestack (there is no plan to deal with agricultural runoff or long-range transport of pollutants); and the belief that the only important harm is to humans and then only if in a form that comes to the attention of clinicians. So in the final analysis, the ecosystem approach the Canadian and United States governments are taking into the 1990s does not meet Brundtland's criterion of a new approach to solve environmental problems. It is a clean-up strategy awkwardly draped over existing jurisdictions and institutions, each pursuing its own agenda, each with the power to block any true ecosystem action.

Jerry Poje of the National Wildlife Federation, a Washington-based conservation group, summed it up when he said: 'the nation's program for controlling toxic pollution has failed.'[15]

12

The New Public Health: A Change in Attitude

The Roman Empire is said to have started its downward slide to extinction when the accumulated effects of traces of lead in their food and drink caused the mental decline of its leaders. The point of this theory is that it was not a case of isolated poisonings; the entire upper class was exposed to lead from its pewter cooking vessels, vessels which only the wealthy could afford. Nor was it a case of the Romans being unaware of lead poisoning: as early as the first century BC Vitruvius, a skilled engineer, noting the sickly pallor of those who worked with lead, warned against drinking water from lead pipes. But the Romans seemed to take no heed or be unaware of the harmful effect of long-term exposure to lead which, accumulating in small amounts in the brain, has a similar effect to that of a drop of molasses in a wrist watch. The brain continues to run, but sluggishly. If the theory is correct, it must have been one of the earliest cases of a whole group of people succumbing to the adverse effects of toxins in their environment.

The Roman tale would also be one of the earliest examples of a massive failure in public health. And here we define public health in its broadest sense: the impact of any aspect of the environment on human populations. We have to ask if today's authorities are any better than the ancient Romans in recognizing and doing something about public health problems. The answer is yes and no. We understand better the effect on human health of toxic agents, whether they be bacteria or chemicals, but, paradoxically, we seem as unskilful as the Romans in actually protecting the population from adverse environmental effects. So the question is not simply one of understanding; it is one of having the institutions and authority to drive the protection.

We seem unable to get our environmental act together and create the necessary institutions and authority. On one hand we have environmentalists detailing the downward slide of the earth's ecology; on the other hand we have the health authorities who fail to see the slide. The health-care system by its institutional nature is not equipped to look outward at the environmental causes of human affliction. And yet – and here is the paradox – it is the authorities of that system (the doctors, the medical–industrial leaders, the health bureaucrats) who determine what is and what is not an environmental threat to health. It is they who sit in the driver's seat when it comes to making and applying environmental policy.

It is accurate to say that this dominance directs environmental thinking in a narrow channel that discourages taking a broader view of environmental impacts. We tend to look at each impact in isolation, asking, for example, if we dump waste or destroy a wetland, does it pose a threat to our health? If medical authorities, according to their criteria, say yes, then we consider regulating the impact (or we may say the harm is acceptable because of economic tradeoffs). In other words, we identify a health hazard and a connecting curative action. The irony of relying on medical criteria is that, for the most part, authorities are unable to connect health hazards with specific environmental threats. The result: public motivation for action is undercut.

The opposite of this approach, the preventive mode, is less concerned with waiting to identify specific evidence of cause-and-effect links. Very simply, we say: we do not know exactly what effect any environmental impact has on our health so we do not dump toxic wastes, for example, or destroy ecosystems – period.

In this final chapter, I plan to deal with the question of how to bring about the switch to prevention. It will not be an easy question to address, because the switch demands a hairpin turn in the direction of environmental policy-making and enters an uncharted realm of social change. It is a monumental undertaking in which we turn around basic attitudes of our whole industrial society. To make the turn, I see four requirements: (1) drop the cause-and-effect thinking (biomedical model) of medical authority; (2) think in terms of relieving the pressure on the environment; (3) design new approaches for learning how to apply preventive action; (4) project the eventual payoff of preventive action farther into the future than we are used to doing.

Before dealing with each requirement in turn, let me repeat that what we are concerned with is how government, business and other institutions *act* towards the environment, not with what they *say* they are going to do. It is these collective attitudes and actions (or inactions) that determine our response to environmental ills. That is not to say individuals in government or business may not show more insight than is reflected in collective actions. Senator Albert Gore Jr, for one, expresses his unhappiness with attitudes within his government and within the business world and he challenges government and business to make the hairpin turn. In his words: 'Humankind has suddenly entered into a broad new relationship with our planet. Unless we quickly and profoundly change the course of our civilization, we face an immediate and grave danger of destroying the worldwide ecological system as we know it.'[1]

The Case for Shedding the Influence of Medical Authority

I devoted the first section of this book to how and why medical authority, in particular, and the health-care system, in general, influence decision-making in the environmental sector. I have done this to make a case for shedding the influence of medical authority. That influence has become a serious drag on the evolution of environmental policy. This drag is not malevolent. The health-care system did not ask to be put in the driver's seat of environmental policy. The fault lies more with the environmental bureaucrats who, in looking for ways to justify their policy, seized one branch of the health-care system as their model for environmental impacts on health – industrial hygiene.

Industrial hygiene covers hazards of the work place, sometimes referred to as occupational health. It deals with mechanical hazards and chemicals to which workers are exposed. Realization that chemical pollution in factories could be harmful first occurred in the nineteenth century, when the first what we could call environmental laws were enacted to protect workers from undue exposure. This experience engendered a certain attitude towards what exposure to a chemical means to a human being: simply, that the chemical has to be known, the degree of exposure has to be known and any harmful effects have to be validated by a doctor – and generally have to be severe enough to keep the worker from working. For the purpose of the law, it became a question of figuring out how much exposure workers could 'safely' endure. Such laws initially were not very stringent and, in many countries, remain weak today. Nevertheless, whether the laws are weak or strong, the idea of single chemical exposure connected to a clinical definition of gross clinical harm, like cancer, remains the basis of industrial hygiene.

When environmental laws were enacted and applied in this century, particularly the sheaf of laws enacted in the past two decades, lawmakers just extended the principles of industrial hygiene to the environment: ideas of single chemical exposure, a demonstrated connection between a chemical and harm done, and so on. As we have seen, environmental situations seldom approximate to what is found in a factory. Exposure is to multiple chemicals, twenty-four hours a day; there are delayed effects; there are effects passed on to the next generation; and so on. Yet in spite of the fact that the environment is not a factory, politicians and environmental bureaucrats persist bull-like in applying industrial hygiene methods to the environment.

Industrial hygiene depends on medical authority for assessment of the harm done to humans, so in extending this approach to the environment, environmental laws and regulations incorporate the same dependence. The biomedical model of medical authority became the operating basis for assessing whether or not there is harm in any given environmental situation.

We saw this influence in the misnamed ecosystem approach to cleaning up the Great Lakes. The sources of Great Lakes pollution are well known: long-range transport of pollutants, dumps, and thousands of point and non-point sources around the lakes. The pollution is measured in tens of thousands of different toxic chemicals and its effects are measured in decaying wildlife. This is all common knowledge, yet the Canadian and United States governments came up with an action plan that selectively designates 350 chemicals as the bad actors (a short list of eleven was designated *very* bad). Just how would you apply industrial hygiene to the true situation of a multitude of pollutants that permeate everyone and everything in the Great Lakes basin? Knowing no other way of dealing with the situation, the bureaucrats concentrate their action plan on reducing the amount of each of the 350 below an 'acceptable' level. Underlying the goal is the assumption that stopping discharge of the 350 chemicals cleans up the lakes.

One of the less helpful aspects of extending industrial hygiene to a complex environmental situation such as the Great Lakes is that public relations becomes necessary to make the populace believe clean-up is taking place. One is reminded of the promotion of drugs. People wanting relief from various ills, from colds to more serious problems, become gullible purchasers of expensive drugs that offer a promise of relief but fail to deliver. The Great Lakes clean-up promises relief by 'curing' 350 chemicals; but it will not, in fact, relieve the degradation. Frankness about the complexity of the Great Lakes stress might go a long way to helping the public understand what is needed to change 'the course of our civilization'.

The philosophical basis underlying the preventive approach is that we humans are part of the world ecology, part of the web of living organisms. Harm to any component is harm to us. In contrast, the philosophy underlying the industrial hygiene approach treats the environment as a separate backdrop that may or may not contain things that can harm us. It is difficult to see how the switch to preventive action in the environmental field can come about until environmental decision-makers shed the dominance of medical authority and its biomedical model. It is indeed a hairpin turn in thinking, but one that is critical to turning environmental policy around and confronting head on with open eyes the grave danger of ecological destruction before us.

I have made the point that practically all environmental laws and regulations have been motivated by threats to human health. With a switch to preventive action, we can expect this motivation to merge into a concern for the ecosystem itself. It should be a matter of common sense that human health will be unsustainable in an unhealthy environment. It is a case the World Health Organization makes: 'It is unlikely a high level of human health can be sustained indefinitely in an environment markedly deteriorating under impact of chemical and other hazards.'[2]

You would think that the health-care system would share this preventive outlook; but on the contrary, the system shrugs off prevention, maintaining an overwhelming bias towards cure. So, suggesting that the environmental sector shed the influence of medical authority means suggesting it shed the authority vested in cure.

There is always the possibility, of course, that the health-care system will move towards a balance of cure with prevention, in other words, show both sides of the Asclepius–Hygeia coin. Many health critics make the point that the health-care system would provide better care for the population if the system became more prevention-oriented. But because of the powerful forces arrayed against a turn towards prevention, it is a bookmaker's guess whether or not the turn comes about. Nevertheless, if the health-care system should adopt a more preventive posture, there is no question that this would boost the preventive approach to environmental protection.

Desirable as a change in attitude of the health-care system would be, the environmental sector cannot wait for this and must get on with its own task. Thomas Lovejoy, vice-president of the Smithsonian Institution, Washington DC, says that the great environmental struggles will be either won or lost in the 1990s. Lovejoy gives us no more than twenty years to turn the world environmental situation around.[3]

Relieving the Pressure on the World Ecosystem

The scale of world environmental problems that we already know about staggers the mind almost to the point of paralysis. We seem overwhelmed by the task of mounting an adequate response. One reason is that we tend to view the problems from the outmoded curative approach which clearly, as we see from the Great Lakes example, does not work. The preventive approach offers no easy road to solutions, but at least opens up the possibility of success. The approach can be summed up in a phrase: relieve the pressure on the environment. Don't demand evidence for cause-and-effect linkages. Unblock the paralysis by exercising common sense, relieving pressures at every level: personal, community, international.

There are many ways of relieving the pressure on the global ecosystem. One of the simplest and most painless is the old adage of doing more with less, but this is not a policy vigorously pursued in the industrialized nations. Take energy, for instance. Industrial societies run on energy; it is the basis for our high standard of living. But we now find that burning fossil fuel, the main source of energy, is driving up world temperature. There are ways of approaching this problem that do not require a big outlay in new nuclear plants and that do not require a lowering of living standards. The easiest way is conservation. Gerald Leach, an advocate of energy conservation, for example, in his report on a low-energy strategy for Britain, calculated that Britain could have fifty years of sustained economic growth using less primary energy than it does today.[4]

Consider that the technical means to cancel the output of 120 Chernobyl-size electric power stations (1,000 MW) is at hand, simply by switching to more efficient lighting. This is what Amory Lovins, a leader in advocating efficient energy use, says. Lovins points out that light bulbs are now made that consume only 11 watts and throw as much light as a standard 50 watt bulb. An 18 watt high-efficiency bulb gives as much light as a 75 watt bulb. He says the world could have as much light as it has now using only 8 per cent as much electricity. 'The energy we waste in the United States costs us more than the $10,000-a-second military budget.'[5]

Lovins points to many other energy-saving technologies: refrigerators that run on 8 per cent as much electricity as current models; freezers that use 16 per cent as much electricity. Manufacturing plants have many opportunities for saving power, if they apply some ingenuity. He cites examples of industries cutting their power requirements in half by re-designing processes. The point he makes is that the technology is available right now; it just has to be introduced into the general economy. Overall, the economy and lifestyle of the industrialized nations, according to Lovins, could be supported using 75 per cent less electricty than at present.

The figure that Lovins cites is over and above what the industrialized countries have already saved since the energy crunch of 1973, when petroleum prices leaped and availability of oil became precarious. West-ern countries and Japan then launched highly successful programmes to make their economies more efficient. Between 1973 and 1984 European countries increased energy efficiency by 16 per cent; Japan achieved a 29 per cent increase.[6] The United States, during the same period (and starting with a more wasteful economy), achieved a 23 per cent increase in efficiency, which amounts to a saving of $150 billion a year. The United States' saving in fuel alone is the equivalent of five supertankers arriving at its coasts every day.

These savings are hard evidence that the populations of the industrial-ized countries are capable of saving energy, given sufficient provocation. The incentive after the 1973 oil crisis was economic. But oil prices have since plummeted, and the incentive for saving energy now is environmental; in particular, reducing emissions of the greenhouse gases and gases that produce acid rain. Atmospheric scientists estimate that a 50 per cent reduction in carbon dioxide generation is imperative to bring the carbon dioxide cycle back into balance. That reduction could be realized through the kind of energy savings Lovins envisages, using technology available now. This solution would also avoid the switch from coal-fired electric power plants to nuclear power plants advocated by the nuclear industry as the way to cut dependency on coal.

Central governments have yet to start thinking in preventive terms. The technology Lovins cites has been available for several years, but there is no systematic government programme to move in the direction of energy efficiency. One sees this lack of overall planning, for example, in the generation of electricity from photovoltaic or solar cells. The electricity from these cells is about four times as expensive as that from coal-fired power stations, but its costs are in the same region as those of nuclear energy, and with large-scale use the price would come down. Yet governments have not encouraged this source of energy. The United States, the largest consumer of energy in the world, consistently cut funding for research into this type of energy in spite of having a large section of its land mass perpetually in full sunlight.

The private sector seems no more capable of thinking in preventive terms. Robert Stempel, president of the General Motors Corporation, argued before the Department of Transportation to change the regulation that decrees that a company's output of cars has to meet an average mileage. Stempel wanted the fleet average (the average miles per gallon achieved by all the cars a manufacturer makes in one year) lowered from 27.5 miles per gallon to 26.5, which would allow General Motors to build more large cars with larger engines. A drop of one mile per gallon in the fleet average requires 420,000 more barrels of oil, 2.6 per cent of the US daily consumption of oil. Stempel argued that the high average mileage gave unfair advantage to Japanese producers because they concentrated on smaller cars. 'I don't want our people spending time trying to think', Stempel said, 'how we can tinker with our products and competitive plans in non-productive ways, to reduce the value of our products to consumers just to meet a CAFE standard [fleet average] that creates an advantage for foreign producers without increased energy security.'[7] Stempel's argument about competition and regulation is raised constantly and is one of the barriers to implementing a preventive approach. Businesses chafe at the imposition of regulations and they fight to remove or emasculate them; but Stempel's argument is also an argument by default for more government control. Business left on its own seems incapable of rising to the challenge of doing something about global degradation. George Woodwell, head of the Woods Hole Research Center, Woods Hole, Massachusetts, an ecologist who has given much thought to these global issues, would agree: 'the control of these problems has not emerged from the free market,' he said. 'There is no alternative to government regulation; that's what governments are for.'[8]

In adopting a preventive approach, governments need, however, to avoid the temptation of microregulating. An analogy is the way governments regulate commercial air traffic and automobile traffic. Movement of airplanes is regulated individually. Airplane pilots are controlled from takeoff to landing. Car drivers, on the other hand, adhere to general laws – driving on one side of the road, stopping for red lights, etc. – but there is no attempt at individual control. Environmental regulation, by and large, has been of the airplane type – individual pollutants, individual cases – but it is time for environmental regulation to move to the automobile type, with broad workable regulations at the international level and penalties for violation. It is the microregulations that weigh down and irritate business leaders. For example, instead of regulating each chemical substance in great detail, the overall mix used by a factory or business concern could be regulated.

Economizing through Information Technology

Relieving pressure on the world ecosystem is not only a matter of regulating existing industrial practice; changes in practice can help relieve the pressure. Much of the pressure on global ecology comes from what are often referred to as smokestack industries and their products – steel, coal, chemicals. These industries enjoyed unregulated growth from the beginning of the industrial revolution to recent times. Much environmental regulation is directed at the past bad practices of these industries and coping with products that in a more environmentally enlightened time would not have been put on the market, e.g. PCBs and CFCs. But while environmentalists and government regulators try to cope with these problems, another revolution is sweeping through society – information technology. This revolution is changing the way our society operates and offers opportunities both for controlling smokestack pollution and for nipping new forms of environmental stress in the bud before they bloom.

Over 40 per cent of all new investment in plant and equipment is now going into information technology: computers, telecommunication devices and software. The Office of Technology Assessment (OTA) of the United States Congress found that this new technology is provoking a profound change in the way the American economy is analysed and guided. Instead of looking at the production figures within traditional economic slices, such as agriculture or seafood, managers analyse the interaction of networks of producers and consumers in terms of quality of goods and services, types of jobs, and changing consumer tastes and values. OTA notes that this new type of information feedback creates an opportunity to move away from the centralized economic management and mass production that has dominated the economic scene this century to highly flexible, smaller-scale activities that fill small niches at the local level.

Skilful use of this information, according to OTA, can mean a 40–60 per cent decline in the natural resources needed to sustain a given level of economic activity.[9] That is good news from the environmental perspective; but just getting more value from a given resource in itself is only the start. Thus, while business and government leaders enthusiastically embrace the new information economy, they have to start thinking of how to integrate the economic information with the impacts on the environment. Prediction of such impacts was notably absent from the OTA's analysis. But there is no reason why the new information technology cannot be applied to building prevention into industrial and business practice and heading off new environmental problems before they develop.

In fact, all the problems of global degradation we have identified have arisen from past actions. While we have to catch up with these problems, our preventive approach at the same time should be applied to newly evolving industries and products so that we are not laying future problems on top of the ones we have now.

Managed Resources?

In making its case for global environmental protection, the Brundtland Commission made economics the motivating force. The word 'development' in fact, appears in the title of the Commission, and the text of its report couches most of its dire predictions in terms of what will happen to the world economy. Be that as it may, most people are interested in their economic welfare as well as their health. One concept that springs out of the tie-in between environment and economy is sustainability: by careful management of the world ecosystem our economy can be sustained. Maurice Strong, a member of the Brundtland Commission, said that if a business does not continuously renew its resource base, it simply runs down. Sustainable development prevents that happening.[10]

The idea of economic sustainability, however, makes many environmentalists wince. They share the view of John Muir, an early California naturalist, that nature has a right to exist for its own sake. They say the reason our environment has been degraded to the extent it has is because of rapacious exploitation, and they see resource management as just more exploitation, though perhaps more restrained. In other words, it is management for the economic benefit of humans. Species of life that do not qualify as useful are discarded. How valid are these concerns? Can a preventive approach to sustaining the environment accommodate a managed ecology?

The answer is no or yes depending on how you define resource management. Agroforestry is a case in point, an example that captures the economic ideal of a managed ecology. Sweden seems to be leading the way here. Its Forest Management Act, passed in 1980, affects 57 per cent of the country's land area and a large chunk of the Swedish economy; forest products – pulp, newsprint and lumber – provide half of the country's net exports. The new policy is to manage the forest areas in such a way as to keep timber flowing to Swedish mills to allow them to run at full capacity.

Here is how Swedish agroforestry works in practice. It copies the monocropping of modern intensive agriculture. As mature, mixed stands of timber are harvested by clear cutting – everything standing is cut down – the cleared areas are reseeded with fast-growing trees, including the lodgepole pine, a native of the western United States. The lodgepole replaces two native trees, the Scotch pine and the Norway spruce (a favourite Christmas tree). Recently the lodgepole has been attacked by a fungus and Swedish foresters are in a quandary about what should be done. But the fungus is perceived as a technical problem, a blip in the management programme, and does not alter the policy of substituting a border-to-border monoforest for the natural forest of mixed broadleaf and evergreen trees.

Mixed woodlands, including boggy areas, are ideal habitats for thousands of species of plants, animals and birds. The bogs especially support insects and frogs in profusion, providing a high-quality protein diet for the birds. Lars Ericsson of the Department of Ecological Botany at the University of Umea notes that forest wetlands are the foundation of the forest ecosystem, part of the natural mosaic of mixed trees, open areas, wetlands and trees at different stages of growth. Government policy, however, encourages the draining of the bogs to make a better habitat for the lodgepole pine; and without the insects and frogs the birds stop breeding. Moreover, the broadleaf trees are weeded out of the replanted forests by chemical herbicides, and it is only in these trees that the birds nest. Swedish agroforestry apparently has no need of the birds. Ericsson says, in fact, that some forty species of animal and fifty species of lichens and flowering plants are endangered.

Swedish forest management, nevertheless, is held up as the model for other northern countries, and Canada and the Soviet Union are starting to replace logged-over areas with single-species forests. It is a policy that worries some ecologists and foresters. How long can such artificial forests be sustained, Ericsson asks, without interaction of the rich and diverse range of plants, birds and animals present in the naturally growing mixed forest?[11] The time it takes a managed northern forest to grow to maturity spans a human life, and errors in management may therefore not show up for decades. In other words, the feedback takes a long time to come, and the ability of the forest ecosystem to sustain itself may be substantially eroded before corrections can be applied.

Management of the environment in some form is inevitable. But in managing, one has to accept the inherent qualities of natural systems. It is like managing a cat; you have to learn to co-operate with it. Agroforestry takes its cues from the monocrops of chemical agriculture at a time when this form of agriculture is being challenged. As noted earlier, there are conflicting views as to whether the current chemical-intensive farming could be replaced by a non-chemical approach. When you strip away the intense commercial interest in sustaining chemical agriculture, the farms of Ken Tschumper and thousands of other farmers in North America and Europe are proof that non-chemical farming works. This type of farming is still a managed ecosystem, but it can provide food and fibre without the accompanying pollution; and it is sustainable.

There is a fundamental difference in attitude between Swedish agroforestry and Ken Tschumper's non-chemical corn farm. On the one hand, forestry scientists voice the attitude that they know all that is needed to create a man-made ecosystem; and on the other hand, farmers like Tschumper express the attitude that we do not really know very much about how ecosystems work, but understand enough to work with them.

Learning how to Apply the Preventive Approach: Ecocommunity

There are many barriers to making the switch to preventive action: one of them is apprehension at having to learn new ways, of discarding old methods that seem to work. A chemical farmer has reason to be apprehensive in making a switch to non-chemical farming without having a reasonable support system and a reasonable period of time to make the switch. The preventive approach requires close involvement of the participating people. Call it social engineering or social change – whatever name you choose, the preventive approach is not solely a hardware approach. That is, it is not simply a matter for engineers and scientists to work out the technology to fix the world ecosystem; people have to be involved more broadly.

This has not been the approach to correcting environmental problems over the past two decades. There is, in fact, a remarkable parallel here between the health-care system and the environmental sector: both put practically all their resources into technology. The health-care system is dominated by hospitals and the medical–industrial complex; the environmental sector is dominated by pollution abatement technology and garbage compaction. Both health care and environmental clean-up are great social questions of our times, but in neither area do we see a systematic effort to involve people in preventive solutions.

How, then, do we turn environmental management into environmental co-operation, in a way that draws people into its design? I have already mentioned the need for government planning and policy-making in a comprehensive manner, but by the same token, government should not be expected to hand down solutions to environmental issues from the top. We need both top-down policies and bottom-up grass-roots participation of people. The objective is to dovetail technical approaches into their social and economic settings.

In short, any environmental management design must include its keystone species – us. (Ecologists call any species that has extraordinary influence on the ecosystem a keystone species.) Such integration of the technical and human factors is not easy, and few social planners and scientists have the experience to undertake such an approach. We need a way of working out this integration that does not convulse the economy and the country in programmes that may fail or may work poorly (or for that matter may be very successful – we cannot know for sure at the outset).

When scientists want to try something new, they set up a model system to try out their ideas on an experimental scale. Operating on a small, pilot scale new ideas can be tried out and, if they do not work, discarded. The small scale allows for rapid trials and corrections and smoothing of rough edges, allowing the whole idea to crystallize into a workable programme. Engineers would never think of building a full-scale plant without first trying out all the processes in a pilot plant. The preventive approach to environmental problem-solving, in terms of social policy and an industrial strategy, is new, and we should not expect policy-makers to implement a full-blown programme in one great jump.

What could serve as the equivalent of a pilot plant for this new departure into ecosystem design? The ideal experimental model would be a living, breathing community. We could call it an 'ecocommunity'. The idea is not new, but it has never been seen as a model for mounting a systematic preventive approach to solving environmental problems on a national and international scale. Here are two examples of ecocommunities in action, both in Scandinavia.

Suomussalmi is a rural community in north-east Finland. It once based its wealth on a single industry, forestry, but over-exploitation and declining markets undercut its economy, and during the 1970s its economy stagnated. Young people abandoned the community, and the future for those that stayed behind soured. In 1981, with encouragement from the Finnish federal government, the citizens of Suomussalmi established a regional ecoproject with two objectives: diversification of economic activity and restoration and enhancement of the regional environment. They set up a regional working group with broad representation from community sectors and support from the Finnish Ministry of Agriculture and Forestry. Out of this community network several innovative projects were launched, such as fish farming, reindeer herding and individual logging operations in which the operators shared equipment. These projects are suited to the local economy but, in effect, they fall into five general sectors applicable to any community: natural resources, energy, waste recycling, education and entrepreneurial initiative.

Susan Wismer and David Pell, social and economic planning consultants from Guelph, Canada, studied the Suomussalmi experiment. 'What impressed us most,' these researchers said, 'was the broad support for the project among all the peoples of the community to solving their own problems within the context of their own resources.'[12] Moreover, the local citizens of Suomussalmi are going about their community development in a way that preserves and enhances the local environment.

A similar ecocommunity project is under way in Vetlanda, a rural community in southern Sweden. The Swedish project, unlike the one in Finland which is driven from the grass roots, is directed by government planners in Stockholm. Their goal is to help the local people learn for themselves how best to develop their community without destroying the environment for short-term profit. Instead, they would blend the human economy with the natural economy.

Mauri Nygard, a planner from the Finnish project, said of the Suomussalmi and Vetlanda projects: 'They imply an alteration in the scale of values of people in the western world. If the projects succeed, they will have shown that a growth-oriented society is possible, at least on a small scale, in the context of a harmonious relationship between man and nature.'[13]

Both the Finnish and Swedish projects are located in rural areas, but there is no reason to believe that the idea would not work in urban settings. The key to defining a community is a setting of such size and geography that the residents feel a sense of sharing this space and of sinking or floating together. Community planning, of course, is not new. But much of it is top-down, carried out by professional planners or bureaucrats. Such planning is often resisted; there is resentment of what many people see as heavy-footed government interference in their community life. One expression of the resentment is the fierce NIMBY (Not In My Backyard) movement that hampers the building of new waste dumps and chemical disposal incinerators. The NIMBY syndrome, however, can become a positive force when the grass roots are involved at all stages of plannning, for example, as happened in Burlington, Vermont (population 30,000). 'Burlington has one of the lowest unemployment rates and just tied for the honor of being named the nation's best city in which to live and work,' writes Joan Beauchemin, an active Nimbyite of that city. 'That points to a dynamic process that belies the threat that Nimbys will cause paralysis.'[14]

The Green Bay Remedial Action Plan is a form of a ecocommunity project designed to avoid the NIMBY syndrome by involving local people in environmental action, but it has the very limited objective of reducing the pollution from 350 designated chemicals. Moreover, the RAP is just a technical fix added on to the community economy: it is not intended to take the next step, which is to integrate all aspects of community life into a harmonious relation between man and nature.

It is also difficult to see this integration in the Los Angeles anti-smog plan. Hailed as the boldest attempt ever to change a whole city's behaviour, the plan centres on curbing both vehicle emissions and numerous other gaseous emissions, from underarm deodorant spray-cans to corner dry-cleaning shops. The plan is top-down, however, and already is generating much opposition. One health expert and opponent of the plan said that Los Angeles air pollution is not all that bad; it only knocks about two months off one's expected life span. In any event, the success of such top–down planning depends on the fortitude of the planners and political leaders as against the resistance of the affected population to change. A lot of energy is expended in the struggle that could be better spent on working out co-operative ways to achieve goals in which everyone shares.

The critical need to involve people in decision-making is akin to the management of large companies. Many of the less-than-successful ones practise a top–down management style with relatively little feedback from the workers and lower-level managers. Most successful ones encourage a great deal of freedom of thought and action at the lower levels. Big Japanese companies, held up as models of corporate success, involve all their employees in the evolution of the company. For instance, Sony took an expensive prototype of a video cassette recorder and over a fifteen-year period reduced its manufacturing costs to less than 1 per cent of the original. It was the first company to produce a consumer VCR. The incremental efforts of its production employees and engineering staff are what enabled Sony to do what no other company in the world was able to do.

The adjustment of human society to the natural world is going to be an incremental process, a process of trial and error, a process of repeating the idea, each time making it work a little bit better. I referred to ecocommunity as a pilot project, and indeed the initial ones can be looked upon as models for the evolution of workable ideas applicable to other communities. But the concept of ecocommunity needs to be built into all communities as a continuing principle.

Environmentalists often use the slogan: 'think globally, act locally'. The Scandinavian ecocommunities established networks of local business people, industry representatives, community organizations and individuals who launched specific projects under the umbrella of the ecocommunity project. The community network has two advantages that propels it into a higher orbit of planning. First, it creates, as the name implies, a network of linkages between all such initiatives. Secondly, all the information developed in the network is freely shared with all citizens of the community. The experience of the Scandinavian ecocommunities is that their grass-roots networks are a creative source of new ideas and are absolutely essential to making the disparate parts of their ecocommunity projects mesh smoothly. In effect, it is the preventive approach in action.

Timeframe: A Human Half Life

We are talking here of making significant shifts in mindsets, how we think we should approach issues of environmental degradation. In adopting a preventive approach, one mindset we need to shift is timeframe. Colin Clark, a mathematician at the University of British Columbia who studies the interplay between economic and biological factors, summed up the timeframe issue thus: 'Politicians, like industrial corporations, themselves always operate on a very limited view of the future.' Clark added that we will be unable to solve environmental problems if we think of the problems in the conventional timeframe of a few months or years.[15]

When you try to correct an existing environmental problem you work on an immediate timescale; but to prevent future problems from arising, actions taken now may not pay off until far into the future. This open-ended payoff runs counter to the thinking of most decision-makers. Business leaders commonly make decisions based on a yearly profit. Government leaders often do not think beyond winning the next election. The whole curative health-care system operates on the basis that cure can be realized in short order.

Natural systems do not work on such short timescales. Our own bodies, for instance, may not respond to abuse for decades. Whether or not the Swedish forest management plan results in an ecodisaster may not be known for a century. The point is, actions taken now can affect an ecosystem, adversely or beneficially, decades later – whether that ecosystem is a lake or a forest or your body.

So how do we translate this lag into a human scale, that is, put action and payoff into a reasonable timeframe? How about taking one half of a human life – about thirty-five years – and using that as a scale on which to measure actions? If our environmental policy-makers thought in terms of such a timeframe, there would not be such reluctance to invest in preventive measures. Actions taken today to improve the quality of the natural environment in terms of better public health may well not pay off for thirty or forty years, but if our timeframe is thirty-five years then such investment becomes thinkable.

It is indeed a leap in mindset from the norm of decision-making. Decision-makers, instead of making decisions that are expected to pay off within the tenure of the person making the decision, will make decisions that benefit those humans coming along. The toddlers of today will be raising families and be in the early part of their careers in year 2025. If we cannot make decisions with payoffs that far ahead, then hopes of reversing the downward slide of the global ecosystem will ebb and Brundtland's direst predictions about the fate of the earth and the human race will come to pass.

That fate need not be; there is a groundswell of public desire to redress the balance between the human and natural economies. But that public support is being squandered on a series of short-term, disconnected actions that clearly do not work. A preventive framework of actions that builds prevention into the way we conduct our lives is the one approach that offers success.

A preventive framework merges the interests of two main sectors: human health and the environment. They merge into what could be called the 'new public health'. There will always be a need for curative health care, but the preventive framework within which human society achieves health will be the one within which it achieves a healthy environment. The preventive framework itself does not give final answers, but to paraphrase David Tracy, a Catholic theologian, 'It makes us ask better questions.'

Notes

Note to Introduction

1 World Commission on Environment and Development, *Our Common Future* (Oxford: Oxford University Press, 1987).

Notes to Chapter 1

1 R. Dubos, *Mirage of Health: Utopias, Progress, and Biological Change* (New York: Harper and Brothers, 1959).
2 World Commission on Environment and Development, *Our Common Future* (Oxford: Oxford University Press, 1987).
3 Thomas Godar, Testimony before the House Energy and Commerce Committee's Health and Environment Subcommittee, United States Congress, 28 February 1989.
4 Quoted in M. W. Browne, 'New tactics emerge as battle against smog loses ground', *New York Times*, 21 February 1989.
5 A. Gore Jr, 'What is wrong with us?', *Time*, 2 January 1989, P. 57.
6 Quoted in M. Keating, 'Limitless Growth, sustainable development is good business', *Toronto Globe and Mail*, 16 January 1988.
7 Gore, 'What is wrong with us?'.
8 L. R. Brown, *The State of the World 1989* (New York: Norton/Worldwatch Books, 1989).
9 E. Goldsmith, Foreword, in E. Goldsmith and N. Hildyard, eds, *The Earth Report: Monitoring the Battle for our Environment* (London: Mitchell Beazley, 1988).
10 L. Thomas, 'What doctors don't know', *New York Review of Books*, 24 September 1987, p. 6.
11 The chemical name of Alar is daminozide. It is manufactured by the Uniroyal Chemical Company.
12 L. Roberts, 'Pesticides and kids', *Science*, 243 (1989), pp. 1280–1.

13 Quoted in R. Ludlow, 'Apple spray poisons kids, group says', *Hamilton Spectator*, 28 February 1989.

14 J. Lovelock, *Gaia: A New Look at Life on Earth* (Oxford: Oxford University Press, 1979).

15 J. Lovelock, Gaia: 'The world as living organism', *New Scientist*, 18 December 1986, pp. 25–8.

16 I have already cited official scepticism about any harm resulting from Alar. An example of official scepticism about global warming is a report prepared by scientists at the George C. Marshall Institute, a Washington DC think tank, which claims that global warming is unlikely to occur and that there is no need to take any action. This view, according to Juanita Duggan, special assistant on cabinet affairs to President Bush, is 'not inconsistent' with government policy (L. Roberts, 'Global warming: blaming the sun', *Science*, 246 (1989), pp. 991–2).

17 World Commission on Environment and Development, *Our Common Future*.

18 Ibid.

Notes to Chapter 2

1 Private communication.

2 Quoted in M. Marien, *Future Survey Annual 1983* (Bethesda, MD: World Future Society, 1984).

3 J. Monod, *Le Hazard et la Nécessité: essai sur la philosophie naturelle de la biologique moderne* (Paris: Seuil, 1973).

4 T. A. Preston, 'Patient-centered ethic sounds good, but doctor-centered ethic prevails', *Medical World News*, 11 May 1987, p. 29.

5 M. Konner, *Becoming a Doctor: A Journey of Initiation in Medical School* (New York: Viking/Elizabeth Sifton Books, 1987).

6 A CT scan (computerized tomography) uses a source of narrowly focused X-rays that rotates around the body. A detector measures the amount of radiation passing through the body from which a computer builds an image of a slice of the body. In MRI (magnetic resonance imaging) the patient is placed inside a strong, body-size magnet. The magnetic field is perturbed by radio waves and various tissues react differently, allowing a computer to develop a composite picture of the body's interior.

7 Quoted in A. Wallace, 'Teaching the humane touch', *New York Times Magazine*, 21 December 1986, p. 23.

8 Quoted in ibid.

9 Quoted in Wallace, 'Teaching the humane touch'.

10 D. C. Tosteson, The New Pathways Program, Harvard University; lecture given at McMaster University, Hamilton, Ontario, 19 January 1987.

11 Physicians for the Twenty-first Century: A Report of the Association of American Medical Colleges, Washington, DC, 1984. Reprinted in *Journal of Medical Education*, 59 (1984), pp. 1–200.

12 Quoted in B. J. Culliton, 'Petersdorf to head medical colleges', *Science*, 233 (1986), pp. 615–16.

13 M. Menken and C. G. Sheps, 'Consequences of an oversupply of specialists: the case of neurology', *Journal of the American Medical Association*, 253 (1985), pp. 1926–8.

14 P. C. A. Louis, *Researches on the Effects of Bloodletting in some Inflammatory Disease and on the Influence of Tartarized Antimono and Vesication in Pneumonitis*, trans. C. G. Putman (Boston: Hilliard and Gray, 1836).

15 L. Thomas, 'What doctors don't know', *New York Review of Books*, 24 September 1987, p. 6.

16 R. Evans, Address before a Meeting of the Economic Council of Canada, Winnipeg, Manitoba, 6 May 1986.

17 Quoted in C. Kelly, 'MDs found Ill-prepared for Future', *Toronto Globe and Mail*, 7 September 1985.

Notes to Chapter 3

1 *Identification of Drugs and Poisons* (London: Pharmacology Society of Great Britain, 1965).

2 M. H. Alderman et al., 'Treatment-induced blood pressure reduction and risk of myocardial infarction', *Journal of the American Medical Association*, 262 (1989), pp. 920–4.

3 R. Stamler et al., 'Nutritional therapy for high blood pressure', *Journal of the American Medical Association*, 257 (1987), pp. 1484–91.

4 S. C. Stinson, 'Drug industry steps up fight against heart disease', *Chemical and Engineering News*, 3 October 1988, pp. 35–70.

5 H. D. Walker, *Market Power and Price Levels in the Ethical Drug Industry* (Bloomington, Indiana: Indiana University Press, 1971).

6 D. M. Davies, 'The dissemination of information', in D. M. Davies, ed., *Adverse Drug Reaction* (Edinburgh: Churchill Livingstone, 1972).

7 J. Lexchin, 'Is anyone reading the fine print?', *Toronto Globe and Mail*, 20 March 1989.

8 A. Adams, 'World drugs and the profit addiction', *New Scientist*, 23 May 1985, pp. 34–7.

9 F. Lesser, 'Drug firms admit that adverts mislead', *New Scientist*, 2 May 1985, p. 8.

10 T. Lewin, 'Drug makers fighting back against advance of generics', *New York Times*, 28 July 1987.

11 L. McQuaid, 'MDs using Squibb drug in study receive computers for office use', *Toronto Globe and Mail*, 15 December 1988.

12 B.L. Lee, 'Antibiotics overprescribed, local doctor advises', *Hamilton Spectator*, 7 November 1987.

13 M.L. Zoller, 'Antibiotic options: growing in number and complexity', *Medical World News*, 23 March 1987, pp. 36–56.

14 J. Miller, *The Body in Question* (New York: Random House, 1978).

15 One billion is defined as one thousand million, 1,000,000,000.

16 C. Baum et al., 'Prescription drug use in 1984 and changes over time', *Medical Care*, 26 (1988), pp. 105–14.

17 B. Medd, in an advertisement published by Hoffman-La Roche in *Journal of the American Medical Association*, 256 (1986), p.2583.

18 Now SmithKline and Beecham.

19 Quoted in G. Kolata, 'Companies search for next $1 billion drug', *New York Times*, 28 November 1988.
20 Quoted in G. Block 'Merck's medicine man', *Time*, 22 February 1988, pp. 36–7.
21 A. M. Brandt, 'The syphilis epidemic and its relation to AIDS', *Science*, 239 (1988), pp. 375–80.
22 E. Caplan, Lecture to McMaster University Medical School, Hamilton, Ontario, 4 October 1988.
23 Editorial, 'Medication for the elderly', *Journal of the Royal College of Physicians*, 18 (1984), pp. 7–17.
24 D. Callahan, 'Rethinking health care for the aged', *New York Times*, 25 September 1987.
25 T. McKeown, *The Modern Rise of Populations*, (New York: Academic Press, 1976).

Notes to Chapter 4

1 S. Wohl, *The Medical-Industrial Complex* (New York: Harmony Books/ Crown Publishers, 1984).
2 Ibid., p. 86.
3 Editorial, 'World health: a dream deferred', *Hospital Practice*, 15 June 1987, pp. 257–302.
4 J. A. Califano Jr, *America's Health-care Revolution: Who Lives? Who Dies? Who Pays?* (New York: Random House, 1986).
5 D. Hellerstein, 'The slow costly death of Mrs. K--', *Harpers*, 268 (1984), pp. 84–9.
6 Quoted in J. Johnson, 'Children's health seen as declining', *New York Times*, 3 March 1989.
7 Quoted in C. McLaren., 'Overworked nurses say "enough is enough"', *Toronto Globe and Mail*, 29 July 1989.
8 A. Wildavsky, 'Doing better and feeling worse: the political pathology of health policy', in J. H. Knowles, ed., *Doing Better and Feeling Worse: Health in the United States* (New York: Norton, 1977).
9 M. Winerip, 'Waging a war on the morass of Medicare', *New York Times*, 5 July 1988.
10 P. Starr, *The Social Transformation of American Medicine* (New York: Basic Books, 1982).
11 R. G. Evans, 'The spurious dilemma: reconciling medical progress and cost control', *Health Matrix*, 1 (1986), pp. 25–34; R. G. Evans, *Strained Mercy: The Economics of Canadian Health Care* (Stoneham, Mass., Butterworth, 1984).
12 Editorial, '$400 births that cost $400,000', *New York Times*, 22 August 1988. (Low birth-weight is defined as 5.8 lb (2.63 kg) or less at birth.)
13 J. A. Califano Jr, 'The health-care chaos', *New York Times Magazine*, 20 March 1988, pp. 44–57; J. A. Califano Jr, 'Billions blown on health', *New York Times*, 12 April 1989.
14 S. Lohr, 'British health service faces a crisis in funds and delays', *New York Times*, 7 August 1988, p. 1.

15 Royal College of General Practitioners, *Trends in General Practice, 1977* (London).
16 J. R. Hollingsworth, *A Political Economy of Medicine: Great Britain and the United States* (Baltimore: Johns Hopkins University Press, 1986).
17 H. J. Aaron and W. B. Schwartz, *The Painful Prescription: Rationing of Hospital Care* (Washington DC: Brookings Institution, 1984).
18 Lohr,'British health service faces a crisis'.
19 Quoted in S. Lohr, 'Free-market health system: new Thatcher goal for Britain', *New York Times*, 1 February 1989.
20 T. Killip, 'Twenty years of coronary bypass surgery', *New England Journal of Medicine*, 319 (1988), pp. 266–8.
21 Coronary artery bypass surgery – indications and limitations', *Lancet*, 1980, pp. 511–12.
22 Killip, 'Twenty years of coronary bypass surgery'.
23 D. Feeny, G. Guyatt and P. Tugwell, *Health Care Technology: Effectiveness, Efficiency and Public Policy* (Montreal: Institute for Research on Public Policy, 1986).
24 Ibid.
25 R. Wilkins and O. B. Adams, *Healthfulness of Life* (Montreal: Institute for Research on Public Policy, 1985).

Notes to Chapter 5

1 The Associated Press, 'Lung cancer among Chinese tied to vapor from cooking oil in stir frying', *New York Times*, 1 November 1987.
2 A. Hammer, 'Funds are lacking, cancer is gaining', *New York Times*, 16 January 1989.
3 S. Epstein, *The Politics of Cancer* (San Francisco: Sierra Club Books, 1978).
4 'Cancer prevention: minimal resources must be upgraded', *Oncology News*, 12 (1986), p. 1.
5 T. Maugh, 'Cancer and the environment: Higginson speaks out', *Science*, 205 (1979), pp. 1363–6.
6 There are many reference works on Mary Lasker and her role in the American Cancer Society. One of the best single sources that summarizes these references is James T. Patterson, *The Dread Disease: Cancer and Modern American Culture* (Cambridge, Mass.: Harvard University Press, 1987).
7 E. J. Sylvester, *Target Cancer* (New York: Scribners, 1986).
8 L. Thomas, *The Youngest Science: Notes of a Medicine Watcher* (New York: Viking, 1983).
9 L. Thomas, 'The lines of cancer research', *Medical World News*, 12 July 1974, pp. 31–42.
10 J. Cairns, 'Treatment of disease and the war against cancer', *Scientific American*, 253 (1985) pp. 51–9.
11 W. C. Hueper, 'Carcinogens in the human environment', *Archives of Pathology*, 71 (1961), pp. 355–80.
12 Patterson, *The Dread Disease*.
13 Ibid.
14 R. Carson, *Silent Spring* (Boston: Houghton Mifflin, 1962).

15 Epstein, *The Politics of Cancer*.
16 L. Agran, *The Cancer Condition: And What You Can Do About It* (Boston: Houghton Mifflin, 1977).
17 T. Maugh, 'Cancer and the environment'.
18 Ibid.
19 W. K. Stevens, 'Philanthropist's billion-dollar cancer effort prompts second thoughts', *New York Times*, 13 December 1988.
20 Ibid.
21 'Doctors can't explain cancer case increase', *Washington Post*, 1 February 1988.
22 Thomas, 'The lines of cancer research'.

Notes to Chapter 6

1 mg = milligram; dl = decilitre, or 100 millilitres.
2 'Campaign seeks to increase US "cholesterol consciousness"', *Journal of the American Medical Association*, 255 (1986), pp. 1097–1102.
3 M. H. Frick et al., 'Helsinki heart study: primary prevention trial with Gemfibrozil in middle-aged men with dyslipidemia', *New England Journal of Medicine*, 317 (1987), pp. 1237–45.
4 S. C. Stinson, 'Drug industry steps up fight against heart disease', *Chemical and Engineering News*, 3 October 1988, pp. 35–70.
5 R. E. Olson, Letter to the Editor, *Science*, 238 (1987), p.1635.
6 For a review of how atherosclerosis was prevented in experimental animals by feeding lecithin, vitamin B6 and other dietary elements, see R. J. Williams, *Nutrition against Disease* (New York: Pitman, 1971).
7 Editorial, 'Montana explains how to cook a poisoned goose', *Sierra*, November-December 1981, pp. 31–2.
8 'Kennedy calls for upgrading science of toxicology', *Food Chemical News*, 3 October 1977, p. 32.
9 National Research Council, *Toxicity Testing: Priorities and Strategies* (Washington, DC: National Academy of Sciences, 1984).
10 B. N. Ames, R. Magaw and L. S. Gold, 'Ranking possible carcinogenic hazards', *Science*, 236 (1987), pp. 271–80; B. N. Ames, 'Environmental pollution, natural carcinogens, and the causes of cancer: six errors', in V. T. Devita, Jr, S. Hellman and S. A. Rosenberg, eds, *Important Advances in Oncology, 1989* (Philadelphia: Lipincott, 1989).
11 Frederica Perera and Paola Boffetta of the Columbia University School of Public Health have criticized Ames's approach to assessing cancer risk, calling it simplistic and unsuitable for public policy: 'Perspectives on comparing risks of environmental carcinogens', *Journal National Cancer Institute* (US), 80 (1988), pp. 1282–91.
12 S. Waldman, 'Putting a price tag on life', *Time*, 11 January 1988, p. 40.
13 Ibid.
14 The term now used for Eskimo is Inuit.
15 M. Fisher, 'Soviet, European pollution threatens health in the Arctic', *Toronto Globe and Mail*, 15 December 1988.
16 Quoted in Ibid.
17 G. Bohn, 'Dioxin-free pulp products urged', *Vancouver Sun*, 26 October 1988; J. Raloff, 'Dioxin: paper's trace', *Science News*, 135 (1989), pp. 104–6.

Notes to Chapter 7

1 W. E. Schmidt, 'Iowans struggle against rising water pollution', *New York Times*, 22 November 1987.
2 Ibid.
3 General reference works on the quality of groundwater are: I. E. Pye and R. Patrick, 'Ground water contamination in the United States', *Science*, 221 (1983), pp. 713–19; R. Patrick, E. Ford and J. Quarles, *Ground Water Contamination in the United States*, 2nd edn (Philadelphia: University of Pennsylvania Press, 1987).
4 A. Pollack, 'Puzzling findings on bottled water in pregnancy', *New York Times*, 31 May 1988.
5 Council on Scientific Affairs, 'Effects of toxic chemicals on the reproductive system', *Journal of the American Medical Association*, 253 (1985), pp. 3431–8.
6 Quoted in M. Sun, 'Ground water ills: many diagnoses, few remedies', *Science*, 232 (1986), pp. 1490–3.
7 W. J. Storck, 'Pesticide growth slows', *Chemical and Engineering News*, 16 November 1987, pp. 35–42.
8 J. Long 'House approves new legislation for groundwater protection', *Chemical and Engineering News*, 14 December 1987, pp. 12–13.
9 F. Pearce, 'The hills are alive with nitrates', *New Scientist*, 10 December 1987, pp. 22–3; A. R. Lawrence and S. D. Foster, The Pollution Threat from Agricultural Pesticides and Industrial Solvents. A Comparative Review in Relation to British Aquifers. Hydrogeological Report of the British Geological Survey, No. B7/2 (Wallingford, Oxon: British Geological Survey, 1987).
10 B. C. Gladen et al., 'Development after exposure to PCBs and DDE transplacentally and through human milk', *Journal of Pediatrics*, 113 (1988) pp. 991–5; W. L. Rogan et al., 'Congenital poisoning by PCBs and their contaminants in Taiwan', *Science*, 241 (1988) pp. 334–6.
11 O. Sattaur, 'A new crop of pest controls', *New Scientist*, 14 July 1988, pp. 48–51.
12 K. Schneider, 'Farming without chemicals: age-old technologies becoming state of art', *New York Times*, 23 August 1987.
13 Ibid.
14 Editorial, 'The case for organic agriculture', *The Living Earth*, October–December 1988, pp. 20–1.
15 Advertisement: Our food supply is safe, *New York Times*, 5 April 1989, p. 13.

Notes to Chapter 8

1 S. Greenhouse, 'From North Sea to Greek Isles, Europe's beaches suffer too', *New York Times*, 8 August 1988.
2 Ibid.
3 Ibid.

4   S. Lohr, 'Canine virus tied to seal deaths', *New York Times*, 30 August 1988.

5   D. Dickson, 'Mystery disease strikes Europe's seals', *Science*, 241 (1988), pp. 893–5. For a general background, see J. H. Dean, M. J. Murray and E. C. Ward, 'Toxic responses of the immune system', in J. Doull, C. D. Klaassen and M. O. Andur, eds, *Cassarett and Doull's Toxicology*, 3rd edn (New York: Macmillan, 1986).

6   D. Suzuki, 'Some prayer-filled hopes for a better environment', *Toronto Globe and Mail*, 25 February 1989.

7   Quoted by R. D. Lyons, 'Outdoors: bounty of Chesapeake Bay diminishes', *New York Times*, 6 June 1988.

8   Ibid.

9   M. Sun, 'The Chesapeake Bay's difficult comeback', *Science*, 233 (1986), pp. 715–17.

10 Ibid.

11 See Lyons, 'Outdoors'.

12 C. F. d'Elia, 'Nutrient enrichment of the Chesapeake Bay', *Environment*, 29 (1987), pp. 6–33.

13 R. L. Stanfield, 'Treatment of sewage is seen as insufficient to protect water life', *New York Times*, 13 September 1988.

14 L. R. Ember, 'New acid rain study stirs interest, concern', *Chemical and Engineering News*, 16 May 1988, pp. 19–21.

15 See Sun, 'The Chesapeake Bay's difficult comeback'.

16 F. G. Viets, 'Fate of nitrogen under intensive animal feeding', *Federation Proceedings* (Federation of American Societies for Experimental Biology), 22 (1974), pp. 1178–82.

17 M. Winerip, 'Finding ill will in collection bins of the Goodwill', *New York Times*, 4 September 1987.

18 F. X. Clines, 'Tendency of US trash to travel irks Britons', *New York Times*, 27 June 1988.

19 H. Stout, 'The economics of the waste crisis', *New York Times*, 23 October 1988.

20 J. R. Luoma, 'Using new incinerators, cities convert garbage to energy', *New York Times*, 2 August 1988.

21 R. Sevro, 'Monument to modern man' "Alp" of trash is rising', *New York Times*, 13 April 1989.

22 M. deC. Hinds, 'Do disposable diapers ever go away?', *New York Times*, 10 December 1988.

Notes to Chapter 9

1   B. Smith, B. Whalley and V. Fassina, 'Elusive solution to monumental decay', *New Scientist*, 2 June 1988, pp. 49–53.

2   Reuters News Agency, 'Acid rain problem "small, not urgent", US official says', *Toronto Star*, 21 June 1986.

3   Information Directorate, Environment Canada, *Downwind: The Acid Rain Story* (Ottawa: Environment Canada, 1981; J. R. Luoma, 'Bold experiment in lakes tracks the relentless toll of acid rain', *New York Times*, 13

September 1988; *Canadian Journal of Fisheries and Aquatic Science*, Special Issue on the Experimental Lakes Area, 21 (1980), pp. 313–558.

4　T. Spears, 'Acid rain killing 1 in 7 lakes, study says', *Toronto Star*, 24 September 1988; D. W. Schindler, S. E. M. Kasian and R. H. Hessien, 'Biological impoverishment in lakes of the midwestern and northeastern US from acid rain', *Environmental Science and Technology*, 23 (1989), pp. 573–80.

5　'New York study blames midwest for acid rain', *New York Times*, 29 August 1983.

6　M. L. Wald, 'Largest coal user criticizes Bush's acid rain proposal', *New York Times*, 18 August 1989.

7　J. N. Wilford, 'Acid rain speeding the destruction of Maya temples', *Toronto Globe and Mail*, 26 August 1989.

8　Quoted in 'Long-term forest studies offer insight into effect of pollutants', *New York Times*, 21 March 1989.

9　R. G. Lugar, 'To combat acid rain', *New York Times*, 15 August 1983.

10　A. Gore, Jr, 'An ecological Kristallnacht: listen', *New York Times*, 19 March 1989.

11　M. Oppenheimer and D. J. Dudek, 'Protecting the ozone layer', *New York Times*, 6 August 1987.

12　I might add the proviso here that when a government leader, such as Reilly, makes statements calling for accelerated action and new approaches, this does not necessarily mean they will happen. Our concern needs to be with what actually takes place.

13　P. Shabecoff, 'EPA chief puts waste cleanup at top of his agency's agenda', *New York Times*, 22 February 1989.

14　J. Gribbon, 'The ozone layer', Inside Science, *New Scientist*, no. 9, 5 May 1988.

15　J. Gleick, 'Even with action today, ozone loss will decrease', *New York Times*, 20 March 1988.

16　J. Farman, 'What hope for the ozone layer now?', *New Scientist*, 12 November 1987, pp. 50–4. For an account of the early history of CFCs and the ozone layer, see L. Dotto, *The Ozone Wars* (Garden City, NY: Doubleday, 1978).

17　P. S. Zurer, 'Complex mission set to probe origins of Antarctic ozone hole', *Chemical and Engineering News*, 17 August 1987, pp. 7–13; S. Solomon, 'Overview of the polar ozone issue', *Geophysical Research Letters*, 15 (1988), pp. 845–6.

18　P. S. Zurer, 'Ozone layer: study finds alarming global losses', *Chemical and Engineering News*, 21 March 1988, pp. 6–7.

19　P. S. Zurer, 'Studies on ozone destruction expand beyond Antarctic', *Chemical and Engineering News*, 30 May 1988, pp. 16–25.

20　R. A. Kerr, 'Ozone hole bodes ill for the globe', *Science*, 241 (1988), pp. 785–6; Zurer, 'Studies on ozone destruction expand'.

21　M. H. Proffitt, D. H. Fahey, K. K. Kelley and A. F. Tuck, 'High altitude ozone loss outside the Antarctic ozone hole', *Nature*, 342 (1989), pp. 233–7.

22　See Kerr, 'Ozone hole bodes ill for the globe'.

23　The terms 'hard' and 'soft' are sometimes used to distinguish the fully substituted from the partially substituted CFCs.

24 Quoted in J. Gray, 'Ozone preservation called costly', *Toronto Globe and Mail*, 6 March 1989.
25 International conference convened by Prime Minister Margaret Thatcher in London, 5–7 March 1989, to discuss banning anti-ozone chemicals.
26 Quoted in P. S. Zurer, 'Producers, users grapple with realities of CFC phaseout', *Chemical and Engineering News*, 24 July 1989, pp. 7–13.

Notes to Chapter 10

1 Lewis T. Thomas, *Lives of the Cell: Notes of a Biology Watcher* (New York: Viking, 1974).
2 Quoted in M. Keating, 'Experts issue warning on the economic costs of continuing pollution', *Toronto Globe and Mail*, 18 January 1988.
3 T. A. Sancton, 'What on Earth are we doing?', *Time*, 2 January 1989, pp. 20–4.
4 J. N. Wilford, 'His bold statement transforms the debate on greenhouse effect', *New York Times*, 23 August 1988.
5 J. Gribbin, 'Britain shivers in the global greenhouse', *New Scientist*, 9 June 1988, pp. 42–3.
6 J. E. Hansen, Letter to the Editor, *New York Times*, 11 January 1989.
7 L. R. Ember et al., 'Tending the global commons', *Chemical and Engineering News*, 24 November 1986, pp. 14–64; P. Shabecoff, 'Major greenhouse impact is unavoidable, experts say', *New York Times*, 19 July 1988. A useful summary of the science underlying the greenhouse effect and global warming is in the 10 February 1989 issue of *Science*.
8 C. McInnes, 'Newly planted trees threatened, as world warms, conference told', *Toronto Globe and Mail*, 29 June 1988.
9 M. McElroy, 'The challenge of global change', *New Scientist*, 28 July 1988, pp.34–6.
10 P. S. Zurer, 'Rise in atmospheric methane probed', *Chemical and Engineering News*, 4 May 1987, p. 22.
11 P. Shabecoff, 'Global warming: experts ponder bewildering feedback effects', *New York Times*, 17 January 1989.
12 Ibid.
13 W. K. Stevens, 'With cloudy crystal balls, scientists race to assess global warming', *New York Times*, 17 January 1989.
14 Cover story, *Time*, 19 October 1987, pp. 62–75.
15 S. H. Schneider, 'The greenhouse effect: science and policy', *Science*, 243 (1989), pp. 771–81.
16 Sancton, 'What on Earth are we doing?'.
17 P. Shabecoff, 'The heat is on: calculating the consequences of a warmer climate', *New York Times*, 26 June 1988.
18 K. Schneider, 'Scientists trying to give crops an edge over nature's forces', *New York Times*, 1 August 1988.
19 G. M. Woodwell, 'Pollution, erosion, waste, toxins', *New York Times*, 13 August, 1988.
20 Shabecoff, 'The heat is on'.
21 P. Shabecoff, 'Baker urges international action to halt global warming threat', *New York Times*, 31 January 1989.

22 M. Wald, 'Heat may alter world's economy', *Toronto Globe and Mail*, 8 September 1988.
23 A. Weinberg, Public lecture given at McMaster University, Hamilton, Ontario, 13 March 1989.
24 P. Shabecoff, 'US utility planting 52 million trees', *New York Times*, 12 October 1988.
25 Editorial, 'Towards global protection of the atmosphere', *Environment*, 30 (1988), p. 31.
26 P. Shabecoff, 'Major greenhouse impact is unavoidable, experts say', *New York Times*, 19 July 1988.
27 A. Gore Jr, 'An ecological Kristallnacht; listen', *New York Times*, 19 March 1989.
28 Ember et al., 'Tending the global commons'.
29 Quoted in P. Shabecoff, 'Minor environmental gains and major challenges', *New York Times*, 30 November 1988.

Notes to Chapter 11

1 P. Shabecoff, 'Pollution is blamed for killing whales in St. Lawrence', *New York Times*, 12 January 1988.
2 The Great Lakes Water Quality agreement emphasized that the major pollution problem was control of toxic substances and that an ecosystem approach should be applied. The agreement is adminstered by the International Joint Commission, a US/Canadian body.
3 National Research Council of the United States and the Royal Society of Canada, The Great Lakes Water Quality Agreement: An Evolving System for Ecosystem Management (Washington, DC: National Academy Press, 1985).
4 B. Hileman, 'The Great Lakes Cleanup effort', *Chemical and Engineering News*, 8 February 1988, pp. 22–39.
5 Canadian Press, 'Polluted diet altering behaviour, habits of gulls on Lake Ontario', *Toronto Globe and Mail*, 1 June 1979.
6 Ibid.
7 D. M. Fry and C. K. Toone, 'DDT-induced feminization of gull embryos', *Science*, 213 (1981), pp. 922–4.
8 H. B. Daly, 'Ingestion of Lake Ontario salmon appears to increase reactivity of aversive events in rats', *Abstracts of the International Association of Great Lakes Research 30th Conference*, University of Michigan, Ann Arbor, 11–14 May 1987, p. A-14.
9 H. E. B. Humphrey, 'Chemical contaminants in the Great Lakes: the human health aspect', in M. S. Evans, ed., *Toxic Contaminants and Ecosystem Health: A Great Lakes Focus* (New York: Wiley, 1988).
10 In the Visual Recognition Test, the child, seated on the mother's lap, looks at a chamber with two photos. An observer notes which photo the child looks at. Initially the child sees two identical photos, then a novel photo appears in one of the positions. Since the child's normal response is to look at a novel stimulus, the ability to recognize that the new photo is different from the original is a measure of the child's mental development.

11   G. G. Fein et al., 'Prenatal exposure to PCB: effects on birth size and gestational age', *Journal of Pediatrics*, 105 (1984), pp. 315–20; J. L. Jacobson et al., 'Prenatal exposure to an environmental toxin: a test of the multiple effects model', *Developmental Psychology*, 20 (1984), pp. 523–32; J. L. Jacobson and S. W. Jacobson, 'New methodologies for assessing the effects of prenatal toxic exposure on cognitive functioning in humans', in Evans, ed., *Toxic Contaminants and Ecosystem Health*.

12   United States District Court, Buffalo, New York, Stipulation and Judgment Approving Settlement Agreement for 'S' Area Landfill, United States of America vs. Hooker Chemical and Plastics Corp. and the City of Niagara Falls, January 1984.

13   H. J. Harris et al., eds. Green Bay in the Future – A Rehabilitative Prospectus. Technical Report No. 38, Great Lakes Fisheries Commission, Ann Arbor, Michigan, 1982.

14   US National Research Council, *Toxicity Testing: Priorities and Strategies* (Washington, DC: National Academy of Sciences Press, 1984).

15   Quoted in P. Shabecoff, 'Industrial pollution called startling', *New York Times*, 13 April 1989.

Notes to Chapter 12

1   A. Gore Jr, 'An ecological Kristallnacht: listen', *New York Times*, 19 March 1989.

2   Health and the Environment. Euro Report and Studies 100, WHO Regional Office for Europe, Copenhagen, 1986.

3   Quoted in T. Wicker, 'Stil limping along', *New York Times*, 9 May 1989.

4   See J. Harding, *Tools for the Soft Energy Earth* (San Francisco: Friends of the Earth Foundation, 1982).

5   Quoted in C. McInnes, 'The path to the future', *Toronto Globe and Mail*, 15 October 1988.

6   L. R. Brown et al., *State of the World 1986* (New York, London: Norton, 1986).

7   R. C. Stempel, 'High mileage rules may stall Detroit', *New York Times*, 11 September 1988.

8   G. M. Woodwell, 'Pollution, erosion, waste, toxins', *New York Times*, 13 August 1988.

9   Office of Technology Assessment, *Technology and the American Economic Transition* (Washington, DC: OTA, 1988). Summarized in C. Norman, 'Rethinking technology's role in economic change', *Science*, 240 (1988), p. 977.

10   M. Keating, 'Limitless growth, sustainable development is good business', *Toronto Globe and Mail*, 16 January 1988.

11   L. Gamlin, 'Sweden's factory forests', *New Scientist*, 28 January 1988, pp. 41–7.

12   Private communication.

13   M. Nygard, 'Ecoprojects in Finland and Sweden', *Nordia*, 17 (1983), p. 1.

14   J. Beauchemin, Letter to the Editor, *New York Times*, 17 July 1988.

15   J. Cherfas, 'Ecology invades a new environment', *New Scientist*, 22 October 1987, pp. 42–4.

Index

acid rain 140, 188
agricultural runoff 104, 122, 130
agroforestry 191
Alar 16, 99
algae, growth stimulation 129
American Cancer Society 76
American Council on Science and
    Health 120
American Medical Association 59
Ames, Bruce 97
artery, plaques in 66, 91
Asclepius 35, 186
aspirin 38
Association of American Medical
    Colleges 31
atherosclerosis 66, 91
Atrazine 105
Ayerst Laboratories 43

beluga whales 113, 167
Bevan, Aneurin 64, 119
bioaccumulation 114
biological farming 117
biomedical model 23, 28, 55, 183
Blue Cross, Blue Shield 59
Broecker, Wallace 159
Brown, Lester 3, 14
Brundtland, Gro Harlem 3, 7, 11, 89
Butz, Earl 111

Cairns, John 78
Califano, Joseph Jr 55, 59
Cañete Valley 115
canine distemper, in seals 121
Capoten 43
carbon dioxide (greenhouse gas) 13,
    157
carcinogenesis 79, 82
Carson, Rachel 81, 111
chemical soup 106
Chesapeake Bay 126
chlorine bleaching 101
Chloraseptic 36
chlorofluorocarbons (CFCs) 13, 147
cholesterol, in blood 90
compund microscope 27
computerized tomography (CT scan)
    29
Corydon, Iowa 103
cradle-to-grave concept 136

DDT
    in breast milk 114
    in chemical dumps 174
    in eggshell thinning 113
    in Eskimos 99
D'Elia, Christopher 128
Descartes, René 25